NURSE BLOOD

DR. KATHRINE GROVER

First published in Far North Queensland, 2025 by Bowerbird Publishing

@ 2025 Kathrine Grover

The moral rights of the author have been asserted. All rights reserved. Except as permitted under the Australian Copyright Act 1968 (for example, a fair dealing for the purposes of study, research, criticism or review), no part of this book may be reproduced, stored in a retrieval system, communicated or transmitted in any form or by any means without prior written permission. All enquiries should be made to the author.

ISBN 978-1-7636148-1-9 (print)
ISBN 978-1-7636148-2-6 (ebook)

Nurse Blood
Dr. Kathrine Grover

First edition: 2025

Edited by: Georgie Montague & Crystal Leonardi, Bowerbird Publishing
Cover & Interior Design by: Crystal Leonardi, Bowerbird Publishing

Distributed by Bowerbird Publishing
Available in National Library of Australia

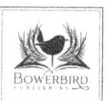

Bowerbird Publishing
Julatten, Queensland, Australia
www.crystalleonardi.com

Disclaimer: The author has tried to recreate events, locales, and conversations from her memories of them. In order to maintain their anonymity in some instances she has changed the names of individuals and places. The author may have changed some identifying characteristics and details such as physical properties, occupations, and places of residence. Although the author and publisher have made every effort to ensure that the information in this book was correct at the time of publication, the author and publisher do not assume and hereby disclaim any liability to any party for any loss, damage, or disruption caused by errors or omissions, whether such errors or omissions result from negligence, accident, or any other cause. This book is not intended as a substitute for the medical advice of physicians. The reader should regularly consult a physician in matters relating to their health, particularly with respect to any symptoms that may require diagnosis or medical attention.

Warning: This book contains sensitive research that has the capacity to upset or cause harm by association with the data. If symptoms result from reading this work, please consider contacting your health care professional.

Link to PhD thesis: https://rune.une.edu.au/web/retrieve/0c966102-bdf7-40d1-9af6-f619385ff0fd

If you are out to describe the truth, leave elegance to the tailor.

Albert Einstein

This book is dedicated to every nurse or midwife who has ever advocated for their patients and fought to protect them from error or harm.
I congratulate every one of you for getting back up when you have been criticised, ostracised, marginalised, and knocked down for putting your health, wealth, and sanity on the line to keep patients safe.

To my father, who taught me to always do the right thing, to be a warrior, to be accountable, and to forever be proud to be Australian.

To my husband, the beat of my heart. You lived through hell with me, and you didn't run away. You held me when I could no longer stand while keeping the Mistress of Darkness at bay. With you, I survived. How lucky am I to have shared a life with you? Take a bow, my love, you are a fucking beautiful soul.

I am grateful.

Just as ripples spread out when a single pebble is dropped into water, the actions of individuals can have far-reaching effects.

Dalai Lama

CONTENTS

Acknowledgements
Chapters 1-25   Page 1-354
Epilogue   Page 355
References   Page 360
Glossary   Page 361
About the Author   Page 362
From the Publisher   Page 364

Nightingale Pledge, 1893

I solemnly pledge myself before God and in the presence of this assembly, to pass my life in purity and to practise my profession faithfully. I will abstain from whatever is deleterious and mischievous, and will not take or knowingly administer any harmful drug. I will do all in my power to maintain and elevate the standard of my profession, and will hold in confidence all personal matters committed to my keeping, and all family affairs coming to my knowledge in the practice of my calling. With loyalty will I endeavour to aid the physician in his work, and devote myself to the welfare of those committed to my care.

1

"Go nursing, love. There's always work for nurses."

My mother's sage words still ring in my memory. I have discovered this truth to be both accurate, but conditional. There is a dark side to the profession of nursing that is never mentioned in interviews or the brochures. It was 1975, and I was seventeen years old. My dad worked with a construction company, and we moved around A LOT. I attended thirteen different schools in my ten years of schooling, had no lasting friends and had no permanent roots. My sheltered upbringing contributed to my naive, altruistic view of the world. My family is everything to me. Their views became my views, and given that my parents were both born in the 1930s, discipline, doing as one was told, and behaving as expected were a given.

This was when the vast majority of students exited school at Year 10, equating the school leavers to being about 16 years old. In those days, there was no such thing as a 'gap year.' If one didn't attend school, then a job was found to contribute to the household, or more usually, the ex-student rose to the expectation of moving on (and out of home) and creating a life independent of one's parents.

I followed in my mom's nurse footsteps, raised on the stories of how she met my dad, a bad boy who lost control of his motorbike on a sharp bend. She nursed him back to health while falling in love with him. They were a true love match. Buoyed by the faery tale from a small child, I fancied the idea of helping the sick. Later, I romanticised the story of Florence Nightingale, a woman inspired to create an army of intelligent women to attend to their patients with high standards of cleanliness and hygiene.

Apart from the inspiration of my family, there was another chance, and influential experience that paved the way for me to become a nurse/midwife. It was 1966, a much more innocent time. Children could spend the day having great adventures wandering the beaches and dunes by themselves. I never remember my mother being worried about me going for long walks or riding my bike. I vividly remember when I was eight years old and on a family camping trip when I came across a young woman sitting on the grassy knoll of a headland at Rainbow Beach in Queensland. A tome on her lap, which I now know is a gynaecology/obstetrics textbook. As a pathologically social being, I talked to her and questioned her endlessly about the pictures in her book. I remember returning to the campsite, my mind whirling with these incredible images. My mom and I often laugh when we recall the moment, I innocently asked her if she knew how babies were born. That was when I announced that I would become a midwife when I grew up. My family laughed and were so proud of me and my newly discovered knowledge. The future had shown its face and beckoned me to study to become a 'trained nurse', which, to the minds of my family, was about as close as I could get to becoming a nun without actually joining an order.

That time of simplicity and freedom was more than forty years ago. I have worked across the continuum of the profession of nursing as a registered nurse/midwife and leader/manager. I have discovered that naivety, altruism, and the Australian mandate to do the right thing underpin a nurse's greatest responsibility—advocating for their patients. Professional nurses are endowed with the responsibility to advocate for patient safety, patient welfare, and improved outcomes.

That is a good thing, right?

Nurses hold a high standing with the general public. It is an accepted fact that nurses are reliable pillars of the community who are inherently good and honourable. Florence Nightingale frequently stated, 'You cannot be a good nurse without first being a good woman.' She also said, 'Being obedient is a good quality for horses and dogs but not for nurses.' I agree with her totally. If something to me is not logical or scientific, I will question it until I am satisfied that what has been asked of me is in the patient's best interest. The demand for obedience and deference to medical officers presents a conundrum. Professional nurses are champions of patient safety and quality patient care. What if, to advocate for a patient, the nurse must speak up against a colleague, a manager or a doctor? Does the same principle apply? My experience has led me to conclude it does not. Suppose an organisation's reputation is threatened or jeopardised by the public release of information. In that case, the nurse will be thrown to the wolves, becoming a collateral but acceptable casualty. In my opinion, damage control ensures public confidence in health care is assured and maintained.

In 1975, long before the Whitlam Government made university study possible for all Australians by introducing the Higher Education Contribution Scheme (HECS), my secret dream of studying to become a Marine Biologist I knew was just that — a dream. In the 1970s, career opportunities for middle-class young women whose parents were not wealthy rarely resulted in acquiring university qualifications. My mindset (my parents' mindset) accepted this fact without question as I continued on my trajectory to training as a registered nurse. In those days, this was a mandatory first step on the path required to go on and study to qualify as a midwife.

I am my father's daughter. I grew up with his edict, 'Do it right the first time, girlie, or don't do it at all.' This mantra was the fuel that fed my high ideals, standards and my thirst for knowledge. I am a high achiever. I started school in 1963. From the outset of my early school years, I would have pre-lined page margins in red ink with perfectly straight one-inch lines on all of my written class work, always heading with a longhand written date with punctuation. Today, that behaviour in a child of five-years-old would be regarded as oddly obsessive. This type of preparation was a mark of an organised, willing student. Standards have been a lifetime paradox with which I have struggled, for not everyone offers the same attention to detail or acceptance of responsibility as I do.

I am a warrior, every bit the hard-arsed, old-school war horse that senior nurses often become; ironically, the type of nurse I swore I would never become. But, peel away the façade and it's another story. I have a heart of glass, which is a huge liability when one works in a profession as hostile to its members as nursing. I am empathetic but scientific. I loathe disorder, so the rigid hierarchy of the profession of nursing, which closely emulates the military chain of command, appealed to me.

Little did I know.

After leaving school, I applied to several hospitals to study to become a registered nurse. This was before the transfer of nursing education to the tertiary sector in the early 1980s. I was part of one of the last groups of nurses in New South Wales to be solely hospital-trained. I was invited to attend an interview at the Royal Prince Alfred Hospital (RPA) in Sydney. I was so nervous. After the interview with a stony-faced woman known as 'The Matron,' there was a tour of the nurses' home, the place where, if I was accepted to train as a registered nurse, it was mandated I would live for the next three years. I was part of a large group that was taken on a tour. Our guide could have been the matron's sister — ramrod straight back, Halls shoes, starched uniform, grey hair, veil, harsh face and a thin line for lips. The nurses' home was a vast multi-storey building that seemed to reach the clouds. The rooms were allocated based on years of training and seniority. If you were a new recruit, the room assigned would be up on the top levels — up in Sir Edmund Hillary territory. I recall the wave of dread as I entered a tiny Spartan cell with its grey walls and narrow single bed pushed up against one wall. The dressing table and single wardrobe were built-ins. A previous occupant had placed colourful, glittery stickers on the metal bedside cupboard, presumably to try and brighten up the place. Our tour guide frowned at the colourful frivolity and curled her lips in distaste.

 That was when I saw it. I looked out the window upon the sea of Sydney city residences, packed tight together like barracks with a sea of red roofs. Claustrophobia completely overwhelmed me! Jesus! I couldn't breathe. Hyperventilating and dizzy, I sat on the bed before I keeled over. A sudden intake of breath from the tour guide preceded a series of disgusted tongue clicks and tuts. If one is to pass out, the proper etiquette is to do so on the floor and not wrinkle the chenille bedspread.

It is said that you can take the girl out of the country, but you cannot take the country out of the girl. This experience was the deciding factor that Sydney, as a place to study nursing, was not for me. I went home and wrote to the other Sydney hospitals offering interviews, thanked them and rescinded all outstanding applications. I was amazed at how focused and fearless I was then. I thought I had all the answers and knew exactly what I wanted from nursing.

That focus became less and less clear as the years rolled on.

Every day, I would stalk the postman, waiting for invitations from country hospitals to offer me an interview. Finally, the one I prayed for arrived. I was invited to interview to study as a nurse at a a small country hospital set in the lovely New England region in New South Wales. Even better, the hospital was only about an hour away from my father's family. So, I was back in the country, close to family and not a red roof in sight. How lucky was I?

The April 1975 intake group of nursing students at the rural hospital totalled eleven, which was a very pleasant surprise to me. I knew the nursing intake numbers for Sydney hospitals could be over one hundred per group. We were issued uniforms, the hem of which had to be mid-kneecap, measured and checked with a yardstick. Also, only black leather polished shoes would do. We were advised which stockings should be worn for the women and which socks should be worn on duty for the men. No choices, no options. This was the uniform. Fingernails were to be cut short at all times, and no nail polish was to be worn. The women's hair had to be tied back off the face, not touching the collar. The men were expected to be well groomed with short back and sides and beards (only barely tolerated) had to be closely clipped. Decorum at all times was the order of the day. No nurse would ever wear anything but a neutral lipstick. Red lipstick, it seems, was a colour that was reserved for harlots, not nurses.

The pristine nurses' cap was made of fabric and was to be starched stiff as a board. Flaccid caps would not be tolerated. I soon learned that the trick was to spray the cap first with Fablon spray starch, iron it (careful not to leave scorch marks), and dunk the fabric in a mixture of cornflower and kerosene. I laugh when I think about it now. Picture fifty or so nurses who lived in the nurses' quarters, all armed with their own bottles of kerosene. Back then, the incidence of smoking among nurses was considerably higher than today. Also, there was no distinction as to where one could smoke. It would not be uncommon to see a nurse with a lit ciggie dangling from her lips, slavishly ironing her caps. It's a wonder we didn't burn the place to the ground. Today, Workplace Health and Safety regulations would preclude using such a flammable substance, regardless of the importance of a rigid cap. Maybe that is why Australian nurses no longer wear caps and veils.

The absence of stars or bars on the cap confirmed to the rest of the nursing staff that we were the 'newbies'—the Preliminary Training School's (PTS) latest recruits, which made us easy targets for more senior nurses. In 1975, registered nurses were called 'Sister,' a left-over term from nursing's religious and secular beginnings. I remember, just a few weeks into our training, one of my group members and I were on shift together when she was directed by a 'Sister' to take the man's blood pressure in bed opposite the nurses' station. I watched her walk towards the patient with the blood pressure machine in her hand. She rolled up the man's sleeve and positioned the cuff. Her lips were moving as she chatted to him. She placed the stethoscope buds in her ears and began to pump the bulb to inflate the cuff. The Sisters at the nurses' station began to nudge each other and snigger. My colleague took the patient's blood pressure several times, looking more perplexed after each attempt. I saw her look up towards where the senior nurses stood huddled. The look of horror on her face is something I will never forget. She stared at the patient with the stethoscope still dangling from her ears. A loud bang rang out when the blood pressure machine slid off the bed and clattered onto the linoleum. The ward was suddenly silent, except for the tittering of the Sisters at the station. The nurse ran out of the room, white-faced and crying. The senior nurses all knew the man was dead and had been so for a good many hours. This initiation ritual was accepted as being completely justified in toughening up newbies for the difficult job that is nursing.

That night, alone in her tiny room, the nurse attempted suicide by taking a massive overdose of pills. None of the nurses involved in the incident were held accountable for their behaviour. The investigation concluded the near demise of the student nurse was attributed to a nervous disposition and that the death of a patient is always confronting for young nurses.

Witnessing my colleague's terrible treatment and humiliation at the hands of senior nurses was my first brush with toxic behaviour exhibited by one group of nurses to another. This was the moment when my loathing of bullying and harassment took seed. I was confused. I wanted to be a nurse because it is a caring profession. I have since learned this is an oxymoron. There is nothing caring about how some nurses behave towards one another.

After the six weeks of PTS passed, we graduated to wearing a cap with one stripe and were officially first-year students. The lessons we were about to learn had less to do with nursing practice and more to do with being socialised as a nurse. Nursing hierarchy is a double-edged sword. Delegation was logically employed to ensure tasks were allocated to appropriately experienced students. For example, third-year students were assigned to administer medications and complex care. In contrast, first-year students (us) spent most of the first year of training in the 'Pan Room,' scrubbing metal urinals and bed pans with Ajax and steel wool. The nursing hierarchy wields a big stick that is meted out to teach student nurses to 'know your place.' First-year students did as instructed by all nurses who were more senior than them, which, in our case, was everyone. No backchat, no refusal, and no going off duty until your workload had been completed to the satisfaction of the nurse in charge of the shift. If she felt like being a bitch, it wouldn't be unusual for junior nurses to be two hours late getting off duty. There was none of today's 'Well, nursing is a twenty-four-hour service' nonsense, where disorganised or lazy nurses walk out the door and burden the next shift with their unfinished work. In 1975, each nurse was allocated and responsible for their assigned workload. It was not an option to pass any unfinished tasks or procedures on to the next shift just because the previous shift had ended. There was no paid overtime. If your work wasn't finished by the end of your shift, then learn a lesson, manage your time more efficiently and be organised in the future. Suck it up and learn to work faster.

The nursing hierarchy also demanded that we stand when the matron entered any room, including the dining room during meal breaks. If she chose to walk around and talk to the staff, our meals went cold as we stood in silence. If the thirty minutes allocated to the break was up, the nurses were required to ask to be excused, then scrape the uneaten meal into the garbage and return to duty. We soon learned that imposed etiquette stoked egos and was often used as a power play, another lesson about the nursing hierarchy.

The first year of nursing training provides a vertical learning curve for gaining knowledge and honing basic clinical skills. This was when we learned to keep our heads down because if we wanted to survive, this was a game we had to learn to play and become good at. Some of my colleagues, fearing more senior nurses, tried too hard. It still makes me chuckle to remember incidents like when one first-year nurse who was particularly terrified of the charge nurse was running behind in her work. She had to make up time to avoid the wrath that would undoubtedly descend upon her. This was when, to her mind, a stroke of genius occurred to her. Patient oral hygiene is a big part of the responsibilities of junior nurses. The nurse gathered the dentures of her allocated patients into a bowl and headed to the pan room, planning to scrub each set of dentures in one go. Relieved, she knew she would make up loads of time as each patient's trip back and forth to the bathroom was negated. The nurse soon realised the folly of her plan when she tried to stuff the wrong dentures into the wrong mouths. I can still hear the charge nurse yelling at her from behind her closed office door.

Ritual humiliation was a big part of teaching new students to 'know your place.' Charge nurses would frequently bellow down the hallways and if your name was on their lips, you came running—fast. The same behaviour was applied to the daily inspection by the charge nurse to ensure the venetian blinds at the windows were all at the designated height and that the wheels of the beds were all pointed forward. If a coin didn't bounce on an unoccupied bed, the charge nurse would grab a handful of linen and reef the fabric free—another bed to make before going off duty. If she was in a particularly bad mood, there could be a dozen beds to remake. To this day, I cannot make a bed without 'hospital corners' or leave the open end of a pillow facing a doorway. To do so was regarded as sloppy bed making, which equated to being a sloppy nurse.

The patients felt sorry for us. At the nominated daily inspection time of 3pm (half an hour before the end of the morning shift), they would sit up straight, like soldiers at attention, while smoothing down their bed linens, regaling the charge Sister with stories about how wonderful we were. You know, I never saw that woman smile. Student nurses had to be creative to get the job done and stay out of the charge Sister's notice.

In 1975, there was no such thing as digital thermometers with single use, disposable tips that are inserted into ears. We used good old brittle glass with deadly mercury. The charge nurses were obsessive about clean thermometers. Each of the glass cylinders was housed in a small plastic tube that slotted into holes (with identifying bed numbers) in a wheel-around trolley. The tube was filled with Chlorhexidine. It would be fair to say that often, the wrong thermometer ended up under the wrong tongue. We now know Chlorhexidine mouthwashes have been associated with desquamations (shedding of the outer layers) and soreness in the oral mucosa. One of my colleagues decided it was too time-consuming to wash each of the holders and the thermometers individually. She made a command decision to throw the lot into the boiling water of the pan steriliser. The result was melted holders, broken thermometers, and a gallon of mercury in the bottom of the metal cleaning unit, and not a mercury spill kit in sight. The charge nurse made it very clear to anyone within a screeching distance that she was getting seriously fed up with this group of first-year students.

It would be fair to say that as a young woman who had lived a cosseted life, I had no street smarts and was easily shocked. There was a man in the Intensive Care Unit with abdominal distension. He required a rectal tube to be passed to relieve the pressure. Anything to do with enemas or rubber tubing has always made me sweat, mainly from embarrassment. All of the first-year students rostered on duty were summoned to witness the insertion of a rectal tube. Oh, Jesus...

Principles such as mastery learning didn't exist back then. Learning was done in the classroom, followed by watching someone else actually undertake the procedure.

Once any procedure had been witnessed, those present were somehow considered competent to perform the procedure in the future. The poor patient was a forty-something-year-old man surrounded by a group of young, bug-eyed females. Before the procedure, the senior nurse went to the pan room and retrieved a bucket, which she had three-quarters filled with water. In her other hand she had a small bottle of purple liquid. She dutifully added several drops to the water. The next thing, the end of the dreaded red rubber hose, was lubricated and inserted into the man's anus. The other end of the viper-like tube was submerged in the bucket. The poor man was extremely flatulent. A series of bubbles, like that from the breathing apparatus of a scuba diver, frothed across the water's surface. Suddenly, violent explosions erupted from the bucket and tiny purple flecks of water sprayed everywhere. Apparently, Condi's Crystals (potassium permanganate) negates the smell of flatulence. However, it does not prohibit volcanic eruptions, resulting in our uniforms, arms, and faces splattered with purple faecal dots. To this day, I'm not too fond of the sight of Condi's Crystals, and that horrid red rubber tubing still makes me want to flee.

I now realise this type of 'training' had a three-fold purpose. Firstly, to actually have witnessed the procedure is counted as clinical instruction from which there was a real possibility that the next time a flatus tube needed to be passed, one of us in attendance would be instructed to carry out the procedure (Jesus, God, don't let it be me.) Secondly, we were taught to ignore the patients' obvious embarrassment, as no experience incurred in nursing was personal. Thirdly and probably most importantly, exposure to intimate procedures begins the process whereby nurses become jaded to pain, suffering, embarrassment and grief. Apparently, a good nurse never reacts emotionally in front of a patient. If that is the case, then as a nurse, I am an abject failure.

In the course of learning to be a nurse, there is a great deal of information to absorb and remember. My first stuff up was recounted around the dining room for weeks, much to the hilarity of the 'real nurses.' What we learned in the classroom was later assessed when rostered to the wards. The nurse educator was a tall, grey-haired woman about 150 years old (or so she seemed to me). Her back was as straight as a die; her veil was impeccably starched and ironed. She had a severe face, but sometimes her eyes twinkled. It was she who told us on the first day of PTS that if we didn't pay attention to our lessons, we would be personally responsible for killing patients. A very effective strategy—we paid attention.

I was required to take an apex beat of a patient, who happened to be a middle-aged man who had recently undergone surgery. As instructed, I introduced myself and the nurse educator and advised the patient what I would do. I was doing great until he winked at me. Every logical thought I had ever had left my brain. I panicked. All I could recall was that to record the apex beat; one had to listen to the patient's heart and count the beats over one minute, all of which was to be counted using my obligatory nurse's fob watch that was dutifully pinned to the front of my uniform. I then did the only thing I could think of. I ripped open his pyjama shirt and plonked my ear to his bare chest. I heard the nurse educator suck in a shocked breath. The man roared, laughing. I never again forgot to use a stethoscope when recording an apex beat. I was sure my nursing career was over, which you would think would have made me more cautious...

The very next day, I was making a patient's bed with one of my colleagues when, like a Globetrotter, I hurtled the bundle of dirty linen across the room toward the linen skip. The nurse educator entered the room to assess our bed-making skills at that precise moment. The ball of linen hit her smack in the face, and oh sweet Jesus, her veil was dislodged and knocked to the floor. To say I was in trouble was an understatement. Not only had I allowed linen to touch the floor (a cardinal sin), but I had also not followed the classroom instructions as to the location of the skip, causing me to throw the linen in an unseemly manner. To this day, I never let linen touch the ground and immediately gave up my Globetrotter ways.

The months flew by, and before I knew it, I was spending the first of many Christmases separated from my family. It was awful. I had struggled with homesickness from my first training day, but this was something else. I felt cheated and so terribly alone. I soon learned that nurses sacrifice a great deal when they are rostered to shift work instead of celebrating birthdays and special events. This fact wasn't mentioned at the interview or in the brochures, either.

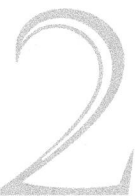

I have always taken the care I offer to my patients seriously. I remember well when, as a first-year student, I learned about the importance of pressure care and the necessity for vigilance in assessing patient skin integrity. I also learned of the requirement for regular rounds to reposition patients to avoid pressure sore formation. Incontinent patients or those with mobility impairments are particularly at risk. Every two hours, the at-risk patients were washed, dried and changed if incontinent. Heels, elbows and backs were rubbed with moisturising cream, and the patient was repositioned. That was the drill.

I recall one woman, M.M., whose name I still remember. My heart went out to her. She had a torturous type of arthritis. Her entire body was as stiff as a board. The only parts of her that moved were her bright, sad eyes. I hated how some nurses treated her as if she were just a slab of non-compos mentis human flesh when nothing could have been further from the truth. She may not have been able to communicate verbally, but her eyes spoke volumes about what she felt. Life had been hard for M.M., and I was very sorry. To my horror, I came back from four days off to find she had developed three pressure areas on her bony sacrum. I cried and cried. The charge nurse took me into her office and basically told me not to be a sook and that if I wanted to be a nurse, I had to face life's harsh realities, of which apparently pressure sores are one. M.M. eventually died of sepsis from those ghastly pressure sores, and I never forgave the nurse who had been allocated to her care on the night shift for those four nights. I knew from experience that this nurse would have slept most of the shift while M.M. sat in an erosive incontinence pad.

It is funny how some events or quirks involving patients have stayed with me forever. One woman was always immaculately dressed in only the best bed attire and never seemed to have a hair out of place. She was from a well-to-do family. When I first met her, she was as sharp as a tack. I recall the day a male nurse referred to her as 'grandma.' She lifted her regal head, pursed her lips and glared at him. "Young man, I have never had the privilege of having grandchildren, and I hardly think you and I are related. You may refer to me now and forever more as Mrs N." I don't believe that the nurse ever again made the mistake of referring to another patient disrespectfully.

As happens to us all, Mrs N. suffered cognitive decline. On one night shift, around 1am, she started shrieking. I hot-footed it to her bedside. She was sitting bolt upright with the bed linens clutched to her chest. She bellowed, "Roll up that newspaper and get that wretched possum off my bed!"

There was no point in contradicting her. Perception is reality, and her reality was that she had a feral marsupial at the end of her bed. I grabbed a copy of The Woman's Weekly magazine from the bedside locker of the patient closest to me and started pounding the bed. After around two minutes of beating the non-existent possum, Mrs N, visibly relieved, flopped back onto the pillows and said, "Thank you, dear. That will be all. Goodnight. Turn off the light."

It is not only the memories of patients that have stayed with me. Sister J. was the charge Sister of a ward. She was also a bully and didn't care who knew it. There was a young red-headed male nurse I didn't really know, who, like the rest of us, was unfortunate enough to be rostered to her ward. He was a quiet soul who kept to himself. He also had a reputation for having body odour. On this particular shift, a loud skirmish came from the end of the ward in the communal patient bathroom. Every nurse on duty, including me, ran to see what was happening.

I wish I hadn't.

Sister J. and her registered nurse cronies had filled the bathtub with hot, soapy water and manhandled this poor nurse into it. Sister J. roared, "No nurse stinks on my ward! Clean yourself up, or don't come back!"

He was crying and was the colour of beetroot. I will never forget the sight of his misery. I guess he just packed up and left. Who could blame him? I never saw him again. The lesson for the rest of us was that we either toe the line or Sister J. would make us toe the line. Otherwise, survival on her ward was not going to happen.

Bullying and harassment? Absolutely. These were the lessons we were expected to emulate if we were ever considered real nurses.

Thankfully, not all of the registered nurses were like Sister J. I remember Sister S. with great fondness for two reasons; firstly, because, like the rest of us, she was terrified of Sister J. and secondly, because her husband died of tetanus. I have never heard of anyone dying from tetanus, so I guess that fun fact just stuck in my brain. She was eccentric and somewhat delightfully addled. I remember watching her through my tiny bedroom window one morning as she hurried out of the nurses' home and across the courtyard towards the hospital. Damn! She was late for the start of the morning shift. Sister J. would have her guts for garters! The more she hurried, the more the full-length corset in her hand billowed like the sail of a galleon. God knows where she thought she would put that on before starting her shift.

One evening shift, Sister S. asked me to accompany her into the medication room, where the drugs of addiction were accounted for and locked away. She opened the Dangerous Drug Register and turned to the page titled 'Serepax'. Huffing and muttering to herself as she fumbled with the bottom ledge of the cupboard, she pulled forward a small slide-out table that was cleverly recessed under the drug cupboard. Keys jangling, she unlocked the door and took out a bottle of Serepax and a triangular counting device. This device is still used today. The idea is to line up the tablets and accurately account for the entire contents of the bottle without touching them—well...that is the theory.

Sister S. emptied the bottle's contents onto the plastic counter when one of the little yellow pills bounced and fell onto the floor. She bent down to pick up the tablet, but when she straightened up, the back of her head hit the underside of the slide-out table.

Oh, Jesus! The entire contents of the bottle of Serepax rained down upon us like tiny yellow hail. She screamed, "Don't move! Don't move! Sr. J. will have us for this!" After a thorough search, we failed to locate all of the Serepax. It was later relayed to me that Sister J. was apoplectic! She reported both Sister S. and me as public nuisances and completely incompetent. Matron was not amused.

I was then, and forever more, have been totally committed to practising excellence as a nurse. It seems, however, that the Fates get their jollies out of having things happen when I am around. One night after a patient had died and had been 'laid out,' a ghastly process involving the packing of cavities and the strapping together of limbs, I was instructed by the Sister in charge of the shift to accompany the wardsman (back then, we weren't so mindful of political correctness) and the deceased patient to the mortuary. That place gave me the horrors. It was in the early morning hours, and it was dark, foggy and eerie. The trolley wheels rattled across the courtyard and down the gentle incline towards the mortuary.

Oh, my giddy aunt! The detachable tray the dead person was strapped onto came adrift. The tray and the deceased skidded down the slope like a bloody Olympic bobsledder. Shit! Shit! Shit! Pine needles and dirt flew everywhere. Thank the good Lord the tray hit a tree at the bottom of the slope; otherwise, the patient would have been out on the road. Puffing and blowing, the wardsman and I heaved the patient, thankfully still strapped to the tray, back up the hill and manoeuvred him back up onto the trolley. We wheeled him into the mortuary, signed the register, put the patient in the fridge, and I returned to the ward. The wardsman used to wink at me every now and then, which greatly unnerved me. But to my knowledge, the 'mortuary bobsled incident' has never been mentioned again— until now.

The next two years were a blur of classroom learning and self-preservation strategies to keep out of the line of fire when, finally, I was a third-year nurse. This great moment was commemorated by the surrender of the nurse's cap and the right to wear a cornflour and kerosene-starched veil. We thought we were the duck's guts.

As part of the curriculum, third-year students were required to undergo a secondment to a local small city hospital, which was a much bigger facility with the capacity to accept higher acuity patients than the rural hospital where I was undertaking my training. The secondment was divided into three one-month rotations to a surgical ward, a mental health facility and operating theatres, and time in the Emergency Department. I already knew from previous rotations that I liked working in operating theatres. To someone like me who loves straight lines and order, the routine of surgical procedures, continuity, and predictability was bliss. I even took on-call shifts for any of the registered nurses who wanted a night off from being called back to theatres at some God-awful hour. Back then, there was no rule for a mandatory ten-hour break between shifts, as is expected today. If the nurse was unlucky enough to be called in and not get back to bed before 6am—tough! You were still expected to front for your rostered shift at 7am. Such is the life of an operating theatre nurse.

The second part of the secondment was to work for a month in a busy surgical ward. The charge nurse was as much a tyrant as she was terrifying. I will never forget my first shift there. I was assigned a patient with acute glaucoma who had a Mannitol infusion running (the object being to reduce the intraocular pressure and preserve the man's sight). At handover, we were informed the infusion must run slowly as severe complications could result if it ran too quickly. Remember this is pre-intravenous infusion pumps.

I checked the infusion first thing after the handover, then went to review my other patients. When I returned about twenty minutes later, I couldn't believe what I was seeing. The bloody bag was empty! I thought about jumping out of a window! Shit, now I was for it.

I reported the situation to the team leader, who gleefully turned on her heel and relayed the event to the charge nurse. The Tyrant came out of her office with the team leader in tow. She marched down the linoleum, shoes squeaking with each stomp, then stopped in front of me and leaned in so close that her face was about an inch from mine. I felt her breath puff on my face each time she enunciated words or syllables. The reek of cigarettes and periodontal disease was truly foul. I didn't dare gag. I am fairly certain she would have hit me if I did. She poked me in the chest with her index finger. "First strike, nurse. Be warned, you only get one strike on this ward. Any more mistakes, and you're on the bus home."

As she turned and flounced in the opposite direction, she glared at the team leader, whose smarmy smile immediately slid from her face. The team leader was clearly in the firing line; after all, she was in charge of the shift when the error happened. Therefore, it seemed the real blame belonged to her, as she should have been more vigilant in supervising my practice. This is when I learned in nursing that there will always be a fall guy to take the blame when there is an adverse event.

This was not the first time I had realised that communication in nursing is problematic. It is all about covering one's arse. If the patient had died because of the rapid infusion of Mannitol, the team leader would have been hung out to dry. The charge nurse would have assumed overall responsibility because of her rank. Though the words were not actually said, the message was clear: if you stuff up and make the 'Sisters' look bad, your survival as a nurse is highly unlikely. After all the fuss, threats and stress, I have always thought it most peculiar that the focus of the incident was on the bag of Mannitol, for no one actually assessed that the patient he wasn't dead, or wasn't about to drop dead. This was when I learned that abuse from nurses in authority is common towards those who upset the status quo.

I was rostered for two weeks to the Emergency Department to get some trauma experience. Well, I certainly ticked that box, although the trauma was mine and has stayed with me for a lifetime.

A call came in from an enroute Paramedic to say they were transporting a young male who had sustained considerable injuries following a motorcycle accident. When the patient was unloaded in the Trauma Room, he was conscious but clearly concussed. Now, as is the way with trauma admissions, the whole body is inspected for injuries, not just the obvious. Both of his arms were clearly broken. The nurse in charge used shears to cut away his clothing. This is something that I will never forget. When she cut down the right leg of his jeans and pulled the fabric away, the leg from the knee down fell off the end of the bed. The only anatomical structure that was intact was the popliteal artery. He would have bled out at the scene if the artery had been severed. Now...I am not a fainter, but on this occasion, light-headed, I slid down the tiles on the wall and sat on the floor.

Finally, it was my last shift in the Emergency Department (thank you, Jesus!) I was counting down the minutes until I could get out of there. Some nurses thrive on the blood and the guts. I am just not cut out for that sort of nursing. Minutes away from the completion of my shift, I thought I was home free when a young blonde woman ran inside the department. Screaming and incoherent, she clutched a swaddled newborn in her arms. The baby was dead.

I had never seen a deceased child before. My world lost momentum and went into slow motion as the horror I was witnessing caused my brain to freeze. I will never forget the terrible sound of agony coming from that poor woman. It was a sound I would hear many times in the future, and it sucker punched me every time. Sudden Infant Death Syndrome (SIDS) is a thief and a bringer of pain beyond which any mortal should ever have to bear.

The third and final month of the city hospital's secondment was to provide us with experience in mental health. I swear this experience confirmed that I am not cut out for this type of nursing either. We were allocated accommodation in the psychiatric hospital staff quarters as a group. In the nursing community, it is an accepted fact that psychiatric nurses are 'different' from general-trained registered nurses. In 1987, psychiatric nursing was a stand-alone qualification. There was no requirement to be qualified as a registered nurse in the first instance.

Back at the rural hospital, the nurses' home was a very peaceful, respectful place, where quiet was required so those on the night shift or studying were not disturbed. The accommodation at the psychiatric facility was more like a frat house! Not for one moment did I feel safe there. The psych nurses engaged in all sorts of odd conversations and demonstrated behaviours of which I understood very little. Perhaps drugs were involved. If the amount of empty alcohol bottles strewn around the place was anything to go by, there was no shortage of alcoholic thirst quenchers. All I knew was that I was definitely out of my comfort zone. My colleagues and I huddled together like a school of terrified minnows on the lookout for a hungry barracuda.

One afternoon, after introducing us to the psych nurses, they all began whistling and catcalling. I could not believe what I was seeing. A tall, blonde man in his early twenties, dressed in a short dress made of shiny, clingy fabric and high heels, sashayed down the stairs towards us. His penis swayed from side to side with each step, like a sad flag; his scrotum happily swinging in unison.

I stopped breathing…I didn't know what to do. They thought it hugely amusing that their green little country bumpkin visitors all looked like stunned mullets. We were terrified and concurred that unless we stuck together, we would all most likely have come to a sticky end by morning. After agreeing with the safety in numbers theory, we all crammed into one bedroom and stacked any piece of furniture that wasn't nailed down firmly against the door. There were screeches of laughter from the other side of the wooden panel, and comments like, "You don't seriously think a bit of furniture against the door will keep us out," terrified us all the more. The psych nurses thought it was hilarious. We could hear them laughing out in the corridor. None of us got any sleep that night. Shitty behaviour.

The next day, we sat on long benches in the sun with the patients. I was nervous and tired after the events of the night before. A man sat at the end of one of the tables, making clothes pegs that were sold to raise funds for the hospital. He looked like Santa Claus – grey hair and beard with the bluest, brightest eyes. I couldn't imagine what such a sweet, softly-spoken man could have done to have ended up in a mental institution. That night, back at the staff quarters, there was more hilarity at our expense when I asked one of the staff members why the man was a patient at the facility.

I was sorry I asked. One psych nurse described in graphic detail how this patient had hacked his entire family to death with an axe during an episode of psychotic rage. The pain and sorrow I felt for that man still lingers with me today. I just wanted to get the hell out of there and go back to my safe rural hospital. I didn't need any more exposure to mental health because I was confident that it was one nursing career path that would never have my name on it.

The torture wasn't over. It was deemed good for our souls to visit a facility for the treatment and care of patients who were intellectually and mentally challenged. A place where people with disabilities and conditions like hydrocephalus (water on the brain) languished, eventually becoming completely bed-bound because their heads were too heavy to hold upright. But it was the child with De Lange's syndrome who, we were excitedly informed, was of the greatest interest to science because the condition is so rare. I doubt this child with the shark-like teeth enjoyed any aspect of life, strapped tight in a straitjacket to prevent self-mutilation. But that didn't stop this poor child from rasping her head back and forth, so her mandible chaffed against the top of the jacket. Her bottom jawbone was white and exposed in places. That child still haunts me today.

The last facet of the mental health secondment was to an Acute Psychiatric Admission Centre. I was appalled to witness screaming, mentally unwell people being wrestled to the ground and chemically restrained. To me, the sound of madness then and forever more is terrifying.

Thankfully, we all survived the city hospital secondment and blessedly returned to normality at the rural training hospital.

I am a bookish type. I was never one for going to pubs or parties. I am uncomfortable with large groups of people I don't know. I did, however, have one great mate - B. At that stage in my life, I had no clue what a homosexual was. He was a great friend and a really good nurse. It would be B. who would take time to wash the elderly women's hair, then add a few drops of Magic Silver White in the rinse water before popping in a few hair rollers. The ladies were all beautifully coiffed for their visitors. He was forever in trouble for sitting on their beds as he chatted away to them. The patients loved him. He was kind and funny and a great human being. He was also a clothes horse. Religiously, every Thursday night, he would bang on the door of my room railing about the latest predicament of what he would wear out on Friday night. Religiously, he would hold up a perfectly respectable piece of clothing and rant, "Jesus! Would you look at this rag! What do you have dahhhhling, that I can accessorise to make me the posh poof I was always meant to be?"

He would then be head down, bum up in my wardrobe, looking for just that right splash of colour he always found. Then he would throw me a kiss and be gone with the pilfered piece of clothing flapping in his hand.

One night, I was walking back from the Common Room where I would go to study. This was my favourite place; it was quiet, with rarely anyone else around. I walked past B's room; his door was ajar. I stuck my head around the corner to find him sitting cross-legged on the bed, clutching a bottle of bourbon to his chest. He was sobbing. I walked in and hugged him. I was used to histrionics from B., but this was different. I pulled him, still clutching the bottle, to his feet. "Come on, let's go to my room.

You can paint my toenails and tell me what the hell is wrong."

He took a swig from the bottom and obediently followed me like a forlorn puppy. When we got to my room, we sat on my ridiculously narrow bed, and he passed me the bottle of bourbon. Foolishly, I took a huge swig, gagged and spat the fumy fluid all over him. He laughed and chortled about how country bumpkins are priceless and that the only reason he kept me around, apart from his access to my wardrobe, was that I made him laugh.

After a few hours and much hilarity, I discovered why B. was so upset. It seems he had been summoned to Matron's office. It had been reported to her that he was overly familiar with the patients and that his behaviour was unseemly of a professional nurse. She told him she considered him an abomination and an embarrassment to the profession.

Later that night, we both sported shiny red toenails, and we were drunk as skunks. He asked me if I had a pen and any paper. Seriously? Did this man know me at all? I love to write! Of course, I have pens and paper! I love stationery. He chose a sheet of paper that looked like crushed linen with purple pansies down one side and across the bottom of the page. The letter started with, 'Dear Bitch Face...' I was laughing so hard, tears were rolling down my face. The letter of faux resignation to Matron was full of insinuations along the lines that she wouldn't know a good nurse if one bit her on the arse. We finally finished the bottle. I collapsed in a drunken haze, still chuckling as B. returned to his room. I discovered the next day, that after he left my room, he had staggered over to Matron's flat attached to the nurses' home and slid the letter of resignation under her door. The following afternoon, I woke very late with my first hangover to find his room stripped bare. Someone told me security had escorted him off the premises and thrown him out onto the street. I didn't even get the chance to say goodbye. I never saw him again, and I missed him for a long, long time.

Welcome to bigotry. I have loathed bigots ever since.

There was one truly significant event that has affected my belief system forever. After returning from the three-month secondment, I was on night shift, where, as always, gloom and thick fog hung heavy in the frigid New England winter. Frost clung to the glass of the windows, making patterns of frozen lace tendrils. After taking handover from the evening shift, I reached for the trolley that held all the individual medical records for the patients on the ward. I picked up one particular patient record, read the entries, tucked the file under my arm and walked down the hallway. The ankle-high corridor lights softly illuminated the length of the ward. After looking in on my patients to make sure everyone was breathing and settled for the night, I came to the doorway of my last patient and quickly scanned through the written progress notes. The small bedside lamp on the wooden locker beside the bed cast a soft yellow light that flickered across the ceiling. The only noise was that of a hapless moth, drawn to the glow of the bulb. Its wings batted against the shade. The patient record confirmed the woman was 40 years of age. I couldn't help but stare; she looked to be a least seventy. The ravages of pain had tracked deep lines into her face, as had the cancer that had insidiously destroyed her body.

The patient lay unconscious, Cheyne Stokes breaths, uneven and rasping. I brushed her hair and then moistened her lips with balm, trying and failing to improve her comfort level. The rattle of impending death vibrated through my teeth and bones. A little after 2am, I approached her room to check on her, then stopped suddenly in the doorway. A beautiful, ethereal young woman hovered above the end of the bed. Her long blonde hair was piled up on top of her head. The neckline of her 19th century gown was modest, although the sleeves were set back to reveal her décolletage and the edge of her shoulder. The hemline of crinoline hung like gossamer vapour.

The air around me was very cold. I watched in fascination as my breath fogged in front of me. The specter looked at me and then smiled, hesitating for several seconds. We just stared at each other. I stood, blinking and frozen to the spot. She nodded to me, then turned, floated across the room, and vanished through the glass of the closed window.

I walked into the room. My patient was dead. But she was so very beautiful. The lines of agony were gone, replaced by the pallor and peace of passing to what I now believe is the next journey of our souls. The Death Angel had come to collect my patient to escort her home, and she was ready to leave.

One shift into my third year of training, the nurse educator informed us that an autopsy was going to be performed on a man who had been killed in a terrible motor vehicle accident. It was suggested that as students, we should attend to understand what is involved in establishing a lawful cause of death. This meant going back to the mortuary, my place of nightmares. Although this was over 40 years ago, my memories are as stark as if they happened yesterday. Remember, 1977 was a much more innocent time. There were no CSI Miami autopsies or television episodes of Bones to assault our senses and desensitise us to vivisection, blood and gore.

I was nineteen years old.

It hadn't occurred to me before entering the mortuary that the man would be naked. That was confronting and shocking, which is completely illogical if you think about it. The abdominal incision was made, and the medical officer extracted the man's organs from his body. Although we bystanders had been issued with masks, death has an unforgettable smell. I would have taken my leave if I hadn't been such a coward by not wanting to look like a sook in front of my colleagues. I had seen enough.

I wish to God I had left.

The man lay on a cold metal table. His head was wedged on a wooden block with a semi-circle cut out of the middle. I couldn't believe my eyes when the attending medical officer plugged in a power tool drill with a small round, toothed blade, just like something my dad would have used in his shed. The high-speed whine of the drill continued as the blade cut through the top of the skull. The medical officer lay the drill on the metal tray beside him, then reached over and lifted the bony semicircle free. The brain plopped with a wet, sickening thud into the sink below. "Oh well," he said, "I guess that confirms it: a severed medulla (brain stem) was the cause of death "

It was horrendous. I remember my jaw was clamped so tight my teeth hurt, and when I suddenly realised the gritty substance between my teeth was bone dust, I almost fainted. The look on my colleagues' faces confirmed I wasn't the only one about to hit the tiles. Someone, ran out of the mortuary with her hand over her mouth. The sound of vomiting followed soon afterwards. This procedure was truly horrible. One of the senior nurses asked if she could suture up the incision (for practice). The medical officer agreed, which equated to one less job for him. The nurse in question was a loud, bombastic bully. We had all learned to steer clear of her. She started to suture, laughing and joking about how she had never been able to sew. The sutures were huge, uneven and untidy. The skin edges did not approximate as usual. I was disgusted. This poor man had been treated with neither care nor consideration but rather with blatant disrespect. I couldn't watch any more. I walked out with the lesson of dignity and compassion for the dead firmly entrenched in my brain. It was a lesson that would stay with me for a lifetime.

Our time as student nurses was coming to an end, which meant we had to learn how to conduct ourselves as registered nurses and accept the onerous responsibility that goes with the qualification. This was also a time for studying for the 'finals'; the exam and subsequent results would determine whether I would graduate as a registered nurse. My textbooks, notes, pads and pens were everywhere I went.

Now, as I have previously said, my family had been very supportive of me and my ambition to become a nurse. I was dismayed to discover there was one exception. There is another nurse in my family who is much older than me. She is also on the right side of the fence as far as my paternal grandmother is concerned. I am unsure whether my grandmother's constant goading comments were meant to spur me on, to get me over the line and finish my studies or whether she was just a spiteful old woman who didn't think much of me or my career aspirations.

I have inherited my father's stubbornness. Taunt me with a suggestion that I can't do something, and I will dig in and prove that I can. I can be contrary that way. This was when I learned that not all family members love or even like each other—a very foreign concept to me. On a rare weekend off duty, I sat at my grandparent's table with books and paper before me when I came out of the zone long enough to realise the conversation had turned to nursing. Grandma proudly regaled the qualities of the other nurse in the family. Suddenly, her tone changed, and she startled me. She leaned forward across the table and spoke through tight, white lips. "And you, my girl...you won't make a nurse's bootstrap!"

3

After months of preparation, I passed all my exams and became a registered nurse. My grandmother didn't congratulate me, and I tried not to care. After a short break, I was invited to interview to study and become a midwife. I have always enjoyed being in the company of women. I admire them enormously. We are biologically amazing. We can grow a child in our bellies with maybe two other children at the breast while running a home, working full time and studying. Forgive me if I am in awe.

I moved to Sydney and started work at a peripheral hospital. Again, I was lucky enough to be part of a small intake. I had grown used to autonomous nursing practice as a third-year nurse. As a pupil midwife, I was treated like it was my first day in PTS again. Some of the midwives would sabre rattle to remind all pupil midwives exactly who was in charge. Sarcastic questioning included, "Do you know how to take a blood pressure? Have you ever given an injection before?"

Now, I had just finished my general training, but some of the other members of my intake had practiced as registered nurses for years. The questions about clinical competence were designed to be offensive and demeaning, meted out, to teach us once again, to know our place.

Midwives are a breed all of their own. They have a highly responsible, essential role to play in maternal wellness and the safe passage of infant(s). I think that, under the tough decisions, clinical abilities, and powers of observation required for this role, a certain type of person is attracted to this arm of the profession. As a midwife, you have to be able to think on your feet, make decisions, communicate effectively and advocate for mothers and their babies. Wilting violets need not apply.

My time at this hospital was my firsthand introduction to the truly bitchy behaviour that is an entrenched part of midwifery practice. I recall my first night shift in the Delivery Suite; it was about 2am. From the midwives' station, a red-headed midwife with the voice of a fish wife rapped her knuckles on the desk and shouted in my direction. "Nurse! Tea and toast, now!"

Seriously? Was she talking to me?

The other pupil midwife on shift was in the group ahead of me; she grabbed my arm and pulled me towards the kitchen area. "Shit! Will you come on! It's time for their supper!"

Now... it is a fact that deference, subservience and obedience and I, have never been well acquainted. The fear radiating from the other bug-eyed pupil caused me to pause, shut up and play nice. We put together a tray with toast and a pot of tea with the usual accompaniments. As soon as I set the tray on the desk, the redhead said slowly, "Room 2 needs a set of observations, and room 4 needs to be stripped and cleaned." Now I know how Cinderella felt.

This was a tough place to work. I never imagined it would be so hard. For pupil midwives, there were set clinical procedures that had to be undertaken and signed off by a registered midwife. A 'witness' was when a birth was observed. Each pupil midwife required a minimum of fifty endorsed witness attendances to meet part of the clinical practicum requirements. A bell would ring on the wards, and every pupil on duty would drop everything and run to the viewing area in the Delivery Suite to watch women, who were unaware they were being observed, give birth. Afterwards, registered midwives signed the witness documentation, and the pupils returned to their respective clinical areas. I thought this practice to be a gross invasion of privacy. It was 1979, and the tenet of advocacy entered my life.

I found the acquisition of evidence of achieved episodes of clinical practice for pupil midwives to be more about arbitrary numbers than about woman-centric practice. As a pupil midwife,

I learned very quickly that it paid in spades to be under the wing of one of the senior midwives. I was lucky enough to have been nurtured by a truly amazing midwife. I will forever be grateful to her.

Each pupil midwife was required to deliver a minimum of twenty-five babies as part of a seemingly endless list of mandatory clinical requirements. When working on a shift in the Delivery Suite, if a woman was ready to deliver, one of the midwives would direct a pupil to enter the room and do the delivery. The woman may never have seen the pupil before. There would be no existing relationship or understanding of the woman's birthing preferences.

Just tick the bloody box.

The complete disregard for the patient and the lack of acknowledgement of the importance of the relationship between the woman and the midwife, greatly impacted my future practice.

Midwifery training was 12 months—again, a vertical learning curve. It was in the last six months of my training that I grasped the herculean responsibility and risk associated with childbirth. I was with a labouring woman who opted to have an epidural for pain relief. In 1979, general practitioners (GPs) engaged in anaesthetic procedures. The patient was positioned on her side, facing me. The doctor was looking at her bare back as he undertook the procedure. I was talking to the patient, trying to reassure her, when suddenly she slumped heavily toward me. She was not breathing.

Later, I overheard that the epidural catheter had fed upward, not downward, which meant the level of anaesthetic was much higher than was intended.

There was a flurry of activity while a mask and bag were used to pump oxygen into her lungs. She was rushed to the theatre for an emergency caesarean section. The baby was born compromised and was admitted to the nursery. I heard the midwives talking about the incident. The doctor advised the patient that what had happened was a possible complication with epidurals, that she should be thankful to have been in such a good hospital, and that he had saved her and her baby's life.

Patients are unquestioning and gullible in the power they assign to doctors, to the point of trusting them with their lives. Studies have confirmed an epidemic of under-reported, preventable injuries to patients as a result of medical mismanagement. Like all humans, medical officers are not infallible — they make mistakes. In the interests of public safety, they must also be held accountable if adverse outcomes occur.

I value equity, truthfulness and fair play and I was naive.

The next event was almost a career-stopper for me. I was on my senior rotation to Delivery Suite caring for a woman who was pushing involuntarily and who appeared ready to deliver. Her doctor was a GP, whom I knew from tearoom gossip was not favoured by the midwives. The labour had been long and there was a delay in the baby's descent. The woman was put up into stirrups. I was appalled and very uncomfortable at how brutal he was when he performed a vaginal examination on this very distressed patient. I can still see the blood dripping from his right-hand glove.

The baby was in an undiagnosed breech position. Now, there is an age-old rule when managing breech births, and it is hands off the breech. The reason for this is that the baby's bottom and torso are smaller than the circumference of the head. This means that while the body can slip through an almost fully dilated cervix, the head of a full-term foetus will not. This is a catastrophic situation.

The doctor pulled and tugged on that limp, little white body, until, finally, the nape of the neck was visible. He continued to twist and turn the torso, then applied all of his weight in downward traction. A resounding visceral snap bounced off the tiled walls. The baby's neck was broken. Jesus.

How could this have happened? How could this baby have perished at the hands of a medical officer who was not experienced in breech births? Who advocated for this woman and her child? The answer? No one. Why hadn't the midwives contacted the on-call obstetrician as a matter of urgency? Are nurses so powerless that rather than intervene in a disastrous situation, they defer to medical officers and allow a preventable, adverse event to occur?

I will never forget that woman or the gut-wrenching sound of her keening, the sound of heartbreak, the same sound made by the woman who had brought her dead baby into the Emergency Department when I was on secondment as a student. Years later, I heard that same sound coming from the television. I shut my eyes, and I almost dropped to the ground. A bereft baby elephant stood nudging her dead mother, that poachers had murdered. I burst into tears as I realised for all creatures, the death of a loved one is unbearable.

How could this have happened? How could this baby have perished at the hands of a medical officer who was not experienced in breech births? Who advocated for this woman and her child? The answer? No one. Why hadn't the midwives contacted the on-call obstetrician as a matter of urgency? Are nurses so powerless that rather than intervene in a disastrous situation, they defer to medical officers and allow a preventable, adverse event to occur?

Today, all public hospitals are responsible for reporting all severe adverse patient outcomes, classified as sentinel events that result from poor practice or system failure. Mandatory reporting of events includes procedures involving the wrong patient or body part; suicide of a patient in an inpatient unit; retained instruments or other material after surgery requiring re-operation or further surgical procedure; intravascular gas embolism resulting in death or neurological damage; haemolytic blood transfusion reaction resulting from ABO incompatibility; medication error leading to the death of a patient reasonably believed to be due to incorrect administration of drugs; maternal death or severe morbidity associated with labour or delivery and an infant discharged to the wrong family.

Today, the circumstances surrounding the demise of this infant would be defined as a sentinel event. In 1979, there was no such thing as clinical governance. There was no counselling for the staff or the opportunity for debrief; it was just, get back to work nurse! The stiff-upper-lip mentality was alive and well. To this day, I am unclear as to what level of investigation was undertaken into the death of the infant. No one asked me for my recollection of events. There was an awful pattern starting to become evident to me.

The death of this infant was singular in the acquisition of my profound professional commitment to advocate for patients. This was the moment when, to my horror, I realised that, God forbid, there are occasions when patients need to be protected from harm. My father's advice to "Do it right first-time, girlie, or don't do it at all" was ingrained in me and made it impossible for me to turn the other way or not report occasions of poor practice or adverse outcomes. The harsh lesson of learning to pick my battles came decades later.

My middle-class working background and family greatly influenced my political views on social inequities and the inherent advantages of the number of zeros at the end of your bank statement. During my training as a pupil midwife, I witnessed blatant discrimination based on whether or not the patient had private health insurance. The situation was thus, uninsured postpartum patients were accommodated on the first floor. Some of the rooms had six beds in each. These rooms were bedlam, jam-packed with six women and six babies in cots. Sleep deprivation was a real issue. The women with health insurance stayed on the floor above in single or double rooms complete with ensuite.

The length of stay in hospital in those days was about four days for women who delivered vaginally and around seven days for those who had undergone a caesarean section. The practice then was that all the babies stayed in the nursery (up to sixteen babies per bay and one midwife or pupil allocated to each bay). It was regimental breastfeeding of the babies. Every four hours, the babies were loaded into partitioned trolleys — similar to long segmented cake tins — and hand-delivered to their mothers. On more than one occasion, the wrong baby was placed in the wrong petitioned slot and was handed to a woman who was not his or her mother. The error was often noticed before the child was attached to the breast, but not always... The babies were then returned to the nursery. However, the babies of the insured patients were wheeled in in their cots to their mothers and were permitted to room in. These women knew uninsured patients didn't have the same rights as those who could pay. Acceptable inequity, apparently.

This practice bothered me greatly, and I was vocal in my protestations of the obvious unfairness and inequity of the entrenched practice. What is that old saying? You reap what you sow. In no time, I was on the radar of the midwife in charge of maternity services and not in a good way. I was called to her office, and she shut the door behind me. The gist of her furious tirade was that I needed to know my place, and while she didn't say the words, she suggested that I was a communist with no regard for social order. She despised me and made it crystal clear that she would watch my every move.

The year of midwifery training flew past. It consisted of full-time work with hours of daily study. There was no time for socialising. I did well in my finals and was awarded a Distinction. Once again, the midwife in charge of maternity summoned me to her office. I shut the door behind me and she didn't invite me to sit. Through gritted teeth, she hissed, as she waved her hand over a beautiful tome that rested on her desk. I had come first in my class and was to be awarded the prize of achievement. Deadpan, she looked me in the eye, clearly enjoying herself. As punishment for my 'socialistic views,' she had decided I would not be presented with the award at my upcoming graduation ceremony. With a dismissive flick of her hand, she advised me to collect my prize from her office sometime after the ceremony. Then she informed me not to waste my time or hers in applying for a job at that hospital as she didn't employ midwives who challenged the rules or rocked the boat.

I remember feeling this profound sense of shock—like I had been electrocuted. Fuck!

My family was coming to the graduation. What would I tell them? I was satisfied I had done the right thing by advocating for those women. Again, my father's voice rang in my head, 'Do it right the first time, girlie, or don't do it at all.'

It must have been the adrenaline… I looked at the beautiful, embossed book with regret, for I love books, and bid it goodbye. I knew disgust painted my face because I was furious — another fucking bully. All I could do was remain polite and steel myself not to scream at her. I was deadly calm when I offered my recommendations for the prize, which, trust me, had nothing to do with an addition to the hospital library.

In 1979, I got a job as a midwife at Sydney's newest hospital. I didn't have one minute of post-graduate experience, yet they gave me a job. This place was like NASA; there were extensive procedure manuals to ensure continuity of practice and the maintenance of high standards. There was order, discipline, and a like-mindedness between the midwives. The other unusual thing about this hospital was that most midwives, like me, were in their early twenties. We were all expected to have pristine uniforms, white support hose, white shoes and an immaculate appearance. We also were expected to refer to ourselves as Ms., Mrs. or Mr. The use of first names on the telephone was forbidden. I always compared the expectations of our presentation and demeanour to that of flight attendants with perfect hair and uniforms.

I had never experienced such camaraderie; it was like coming home to a long-lost family. There was ample opportunity for education and mentorship of new skills, which I took full advantage of. The acuity of this facility was second to none, which meant women with the most complicated pregnancies were transferred to this hospital. Nowhere else would I have been exposed to such incredible clinical experience? During these early years, I developed what is referred to as a 'midwife's gut'; that sixth sense that kicks in, when a pregnancy, labour or delivery takes an unexpected turn and decisions need to be made quickly to ensure the patient remains safe.

As part of our professional development, we were taught how to be in charge of shifts. This was a truly onerous responsibility for such young midwives, and I took to it like a duck to water. I thrived in this environment both personally and professionally and was acknowledged as a natural-born leader. The standard of care was excellent, and the midwives actively advocated for the women and their babies.

These were good times for me. Nurses work hard and play hard. It is a tough job, but laughter was always a part of our day. I still chuckle when I recall working a morning shift in the Delivery Suite — my patient was around 200kgs. She had just had an epidural inserted (an amazing feat in itself), after which she needed to be repositioned in the bed. A functioning epidural diminishes all feeling from the ribcage down. I enlisted the help of a colleague, who weighed about 47kgs, wringing wet in a pair of gum boots. I, on the other hand, I am 5 feet 2 inches tall and voluptuous. Lifting patients much heavier than ourselves is a part of daily life for a nurse, as are back injuries. Dutifully (after I convinced my colleague that this was a good idea), we shoulder-lifted the patient. This means a nurse is on either side of the bed, facing the wall above the bed head. We then link hands behind the patient's back, and on the count of three, we use our combined strength to heave the patient up the bed...well, that is the theory. All was going well until we removed our arms from behind the patient. I got clear just before the patient flopped back onto the bean bag, a moment before we expected her to. My colleague's head got caught behind the patient's back. She was face-first into the vinyl. Her arms and legs flailed like a stick insect trapped in a spider's web. It really wasn't funny. I suppose she could have suffocated, but I laughed until I could barely breathe. Whenever I see a praying mantis, I think of her fondly and chuckle.

This was an incredibly busy Delivery Suite with more than 5,000 births annually. Every day, there would be a caesarean section list. One midwife would be assigned to the detail. As I have previously said, I really liked working in operating theatres, so I frequently volunteered to do 'the Caesar List'. On this particular day, it was especially busy. There were six caesareans booked back-to-back. That meant I had to change into theatre clothes, go to theatres, receive the baby and the placenta, return to the Delivery Suite, weigh, measure and dress the baby, weigh the placenta and write up the notes and the birth register, then hot foot it back for the next caesarean.

By the end of the list, I was knackered. You can imagine six changes of theatre clothes and shoes and caps and masks. I looked like the wreck of the Hesperus. The Assistant Director of Maternity and Neonatal Services was in the Delivery Suite on my last run. She was always perfectly coiffed and attractive, with false eyelashes long enough to sweep the floor. She looked down her nose at me and sniffed, "Miss B, may I suggest you take some time to replenish your lipstick? You are quite the sight, and that is simply unacceptable." She turned on her navy blue high-heeled shoes and left the Delivery Suite. I stood there like Raggedy Ann in disbelief as I watched her retreat down the corridor. Priorities! Clearly, mine were wrong.

A mystery that has dogged me since that day has never been solved. I attended six caesarean sections. I collected six babies and six placentas. Yet I could only ever account for 6 babies and five placentas. I returned to the theatres to ensure I hadn't left it behind. I pulled linen bags apart and checked all the garbage bins. Who the hell loses a placenta? Me apparently, it had disappeared into thin air, never to be seen again.

Nursing is a tough job where nothing is black or white. Sometimes, events occur that challenge personal views and beliefs. It was 1980, when I learned that sometimes when good people do bad things, good things can happen. But the cost to the person is enormous.

A woman who was the mother of three small children required emergency surgery. She was critically anaemic, a huge anaesthetic risk, and just too unstable to undergo an operation. Her religious beliefs prevented her from accepting any form of blood products. The doctor concerned tried desperately for hours to convince the woman and her family that unless she consented to receiving the life-saving blood transfusions, he could do no more; she was going to die. The family and the patient were adamant in their belief that God, in his wisdom, would provide if that was his will.

Being a nurse, I find it hard to condone the loss of life if it is preventable. As a person, I respect that all individuals are entitled to their beliefs and to make choices they consider suitable. I now know that as a nurse, I must wear two hats: one for the beliefs that are important to me and another for accepting the beliefs of others, even if the two are in contradiction. A big ask. I became aware that the patient had been transferred to theatres. I was puzzled, what had changed in the patient's condition to minimise the risk enough to proceed with the proposed procedure? Well, that didn't make sense. I was well aware of the patient's and her family's stance on the acceptance of blood products. I left the question unanswered and returned to looking after my patients. A couple of hours later, I spotted a theatre nurse I was friendly with. I stopped her in the corridor as she smiled and went to walk past me. I am an endlessly curious individual. I just had to know what had happened. We were colleagues, and she knew me well enough to know that I am a vault. If anyone confides confidential information to me, it stays with me and me alone.

After the patient was anaesthetised, an urgent cross-match of six units of whole blood was ordered. All six units were transfused during the procedure. The patient underwent the necessary emergency surgery, and she survived. The intravenous lines were changed, and a bag of Normal Saline was running when her relieved family were brought into the Recovery Room to visit her. They prayed together and thanked God for saving her. They had been blessed with a miracle for which they were truly grateful. You know, maybe they had been. God works in mysterious ways.

I was not present in the operating theatre. I cannot, in truth, say I saw the patient being transfused with blood. But as they say, 'the proof is in the pudding.' The patient survived the operation, recovered and went home to her family. I have grappled with this situation long enough to perhaps begin to understand the angst of the surgeon. He was a highly skilled doctor who could save this young woman's life. But she needed blood to survive the surgery. Could he condone allowing her to die and leave three young children without a mother? The agony he must have experienced when he decided to proceed must have been onerous.

I accept that the patient's wishes were not exercised. Do health professionals have the right to impose their views if it means saving a life? No, but those three children will never know how lucky they are that their mother lived to watch them grow up. The surgeon was tortured by his decision for a very long time; he probably still is. I understand there is a line that defines right and wrong, but to me, this situation was all shades of grey. I know what the law would make of this event, but I can appreciate both sides. Today, I am no closer to having a concrete opinion about whether what happened was morally right or professionally and ethically wrong. I think of the children and am glad they got a second chance to grow up with their mom.

In 1981, I was getting restless. By then, I had acquired considerable clinical skills as a midwife. A nagging thought had been lurking in the back of my brain for a while. I knew I was ready for a change. Perhaps my nomad childhood influenced my propensity to change jobs every few years. I had been considering applying for a job in rural New South Wales. After all, I am a country girl. Being young and bulletproof, I was confident I was ready to work in a small hospital in a country town. It was time to leave the city's bright lights and find the peace of a quieter life.

My family had moved (again) to a large country town on the beautiful New England Tablelands. I took annual leave and spent a holiday with them. I loved the place. It was a quintessential New South Wales country town—cowboys and all!

The decision was made. I rang and spoke with the matron of the local hospital. I laugh when I think about those times. Today, there is a requirement for a formal curriculum vitae, complete with a cover letter and copies of all authorities and legal registrations and then, the waiting starts. After endless weeks/months, an interview may be offered. The interview panel commonly consists of three to four (usually) bored-looking people. Once confirmation of Working with Children checks, criminal record checks, professional registration checks and a minimum of three referee checks have been attended, and if you are lucky (or haven't died in the meantime) after about five to seven months, a call may be received with the offer of a job.

1981 was a much simpler time.

Matron and I met later on the day of my call. She offered me a job without seeing my registration papers or any validation from the referees. Then, she took me on a tour of the Maternity Unit, which was a building separate from the main hospital. When I drove past the building for my interview, I thought it was a barn.

Little did I know, my family would soon uproot and move on to the next contract in the next town. I hadn't counted on that. I looked forward to working at this hospital, where the pace would be slower and less stressful as the patients had much lower acuity — easy peasy. It wasn't.

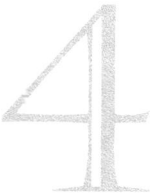

Life as a midwife could not have been more different. I was used to the hustle and bustle of 5000 births yearly in a big city hospital, with numerous midwives and residents, registrars and obstetric specialists on shift. At this country hospital, there was just one midwife and one non-endorsed enrolled nurse rostered per shift to attend to the antenatal and postnatal patients and their babies. Also, any babies who required extra observation were housed in a separate nursery and were the responsibility of the midwife. Of course, women who presented in labour were also directly under the care of the midwife. To say that staffing was a little thin on the ground was an understatement.

I began to feel as though I had been warped back in time. This hospital and its practices were archaic. Seriously, in what first-world country in the 20th century, do nurses hand-roll and sterilise cotton wool balls? What happened to the pre-sterilised packets I had ripped open a thousand times before? Hadn't they made the journey to rural facilities yet? To my astonishment,

I was informed the GPs who had admitting rights to deliver babies didn't trust the new-fangled plastic yellow umbilical cord clamps, which had been invented in the 1960s and had been used as standard practice since the early 1970s. To counteract the irrational fear that the umbilical cord clamp would somehow come loose and the baby would bleed to death, the midwives, as part of their duties, had to measure, cut, package and sterilise two pieces of string that were included with each delivery set. One piece of string was to be tied above the clamp and the other below — a suspenders and belt scenario if there ever was one. This was just the tip of the iceberg of oddity that I discovered at this hospital.

I understand that country folk and city folk are often very different. The maternity unit was at the bottom of a long concrete path on an incline from the main hospital. If a woman was to undergo a caesarean section, the patient and the humidicrib for the baby had to be pushed up a long, steep concrete path to theatres, be it rain, hail or shine. One morning, I was on my way up to theatres for a caesarean section, grunting and pushing a humidicrib that had a very dicky wheel, when I came upon a huge red-belly black snake lying on the path, sunning itself.

Jesus! I all but let go of the 'crib; I snapped the brakes on and just stood there, with my mouth open. Then, a wardsman yelled to me, "Use the stick, Sister!"

The stick?

The look of bewilderment must have been enough for him. He walked down the path and picked up what looked like a wooden curtain rod with a wire hook on one end. As fast as lightning, he scooped the hook under the snake's belly and flung it about twenty feet down the slope. Grinning at the city newbie (me), he leaned the stick back against the wall. "This is our snake waddy. Those buggers are about all the time here in summer. Just mind where you're walkin,' is all."

He turned and walked away. No doubt I was the butt of tearoom hilarity for some time afterwards.

There was one older midwife whose behaviours I found very challenging. Not only did she routinely measure the amount of toilet paper being used by the midwifery staff, but she would also cut the 'blueys' (absorbent, plastic-backed, disposable sheets) into quarters. The women would have blue plastic stuck to their skin, and unabsorbed body fluids ensured frequent bed changes — false economy at its best. It was this midwife who was aghast when, after one of my patients had delivered, I took her to the shower and then walked her and her baby in the cot to her bed. The midwife scuttled off at speed. She returned a short time later accompanied by Matron. The midwife railed on about how I was putting lives at risk and that the patient most certainly would incur a severe uterine prolapse as a result of not maintaining bed rest for at least twenty-four hours post-birthing. Matron, a diminutive Asian woman, asked me to explain my actions.

I assured her this was contemporary practice and that I would never put any woman at risk. At this point, the other midwife started banging on about dangerous city practices and how that sort of nonsense would not be tolerated in this unit.

Now... I know I should have just kept quiet...

Have I mentioned that I have little time or tolerance for fools or troublemakers? The midwife was livid and fluffed up like a Bantam rooster. I will never forget the look on her face when I asked her to "Please explain the science of uterine prolapse in relation to postpartum ambulation." She made a throat-clearing noise, pursed her lips and shot daggers at me. Matron gave a little smile and said, "Carry on, Sister, dear."

Okay, so now I had made an enemy. The Bantam made it perfectly clear that she thought I was a whipper snapper who was too big for her britches. She may have been right.

The nights are freezing in the dead of winter in the New South Wales, New England area. One evening, I came onto a night shift and took handover from the afternoon shift midwife, who happened to be the Bantam. I made my rounds to check on the patients and advised partners who still lurked behind closed curtains that visiting hours had passed and that it was time to go home. The women and their babies were all snuggled down in the centrally heated ward. Even today, it is still my habit to see all the patients under my allocation at the beginning of each shift.

According to the handover and my handover sheet, there were two women unaccounted for. I became more and more perplexed as I searched the building. I found them. I could not believe what I was seeing. Two First Nations women and their babies were huddled up in their beds, which happened to be out on the veranda that was enclosed with mesh, not glass. Frost had already begun to settle on the floorboards and onto the blankets on their beds. I didn't understand. Surely these women had not been deliberately segregated from the other patients, all of whom were Caucasian? I apologised to the women for their discomfort and moved them to beds inside the ward. At first, they were tentative, like children who knew they were going to get into trouble. They finally acquiesced and were both clearly glad to have the opportunity to get warm.

As fate would have it, the Bantam was on shift again the following day. Handover consisted of the patient's bed number and then the relevant details — no names required. Sigh...

When I began the handover for the two First Nations women, she pushed back her chair, stood, leaned over the desk and hissed in my face. "Blacks don't come inside, and they certainly don't sleep in the white beds!"

I was appalled. She snatched the handover sheet out of my hand, turned and stormed out of the office. "We'll just see about this!" She said.

I caught up to her and asked her what the hell she thought she was doing. "I am going to put them back where they belong!" She responded, matter-of-factly.

I stood in front of her, blocking her from entering the ward. "You do that. But know this: tonight, and for as many other winter nights as I am here in this God-forsaken place, I will move all First Nation women and their babies into the ward. You racist cow! You are a disgrace to the profession."

She turned and left the building, no doubt hot-footing it to the Matron's office, which was her standard modus operandi. It was past the end of my shift, but I needed to stay until she returned. A midwife had to be in attendance at all times. The Bantam reappeared unaccompanied, about an hour later. We didn't speak. I just picked up my car keys and went home. When I returned that night, the First Nations women and their babies were inside the ward.

One of the General Practitioners was European. Home birthing was a very acceptable and natural event for him. He asked me to work for him as his midwife and attend home births for his patients.

Now, I have no issue with women who wish to give birth at home within familiar surroundings and in the company of family.

But... I only support this practice when there is a birth plan in place that realistically includes the possibility of transfer to the hospital and handover to a competent medical officer in the event that intervention is required to ensure the safety of the mother and the baby. I believe none of those stipulations could be met, so I graciously declined the offer.

I struggled with the differences in standards and the lack of support in the event of an emergency at this hospital. I guess I was spoiled. I was used to having the best equipment and services at my fingertips while being surrounded by highly competent clinicians. I recall that on one shift, there was a baby in a humidicrib. He required regular surveillance and vital signs. I noticed the 'crib temperature was labile, and despite setting and resetting the temperature, it remained too hot. The only other humidicrib available was the one with the dicky wheel used to transport caesarean section babies. It was about 2am. There was no hope of calling anyone in to repair the unit at that hour. The baby, born at 36 weeks gestation, was about six hours old. Stabilisation of his temperature and blood sugars were the immediate priority. In lieu of another functional humidicrib, I stuffed the baby down the front of my uniform—skin to skin— then knotted my cardigan around my waist to complete the pouch. I notified the on-duty supervisor of the situation and advised that if a woman came in labouring, she would need to assume responsibility for the baby.

It wasn't an option to put the baby in bed with the mother as the child required hourly observations, and the mother was just six hours post caesarean section. The malfunctioning humidicrib was removed, and an updated loan unit arrived from Bio-Medical Services.

A few weeks later, while attending a set of observations on one of the two babies in humidicribs, I noticed spider webs in the corner of the nursery. I pulled out my trusty torch and discovered it was a red-back spider nest.

Crap! I moved the occupied humidicribs plus the 'Caesar' crib into the office and plugged them in, then I wrote a DO NOT ENTER sign in huge red letters and stuck it to the nursery door. I ran the sticky tape back and forth across the doors for good measure. By chance, the Bantam came on duty in the morning to take the handover. She saw the cordoned-off nursery, and her eyes gleamed with joy. This time, she had me! She disappeared with a can of bug spray in her hand, which, based on previous experience, was presumably to Matron's office. About twenty minutes later, both women were standing in front of me. The Bantam wielded the can of bug spray like it was a container of Napalm. Matron asked me to explain. I undid my sticky tape handy work and took her into the nursery. Her eyes nearly left their sockets. Three redback spiders sat gathered around the nest. She said to me, "Thank you, Sister, dear, that will be all. Sleep well."

I left the building without giving a handover, wondering if I still had a job. When I returned to work the next night, professional exterminator signs said, 'Do Not Enter.' It seemed I still had a job, and the Bantam had been lectured on the perils of poisonous arachnids and newborns.

Okay, I had had enough of bloody snakes, dicky wheels and spiders. I was also lonely and antsy to return to Sydney, where professional nurses, midwives, and equipment functioned as intended. I had this mindset that staying in a position for less than one year would somehow reflect badly on my curriculum vitae regarding employment stability. I should have just listened to my gut. When will I ever learn?

I was really fed up, not only with the standard of care but with the attitudes of some of the staff. It was like living in the dark ages. To survive my self-imposed twelve-month tenure at this hospital, I opted to work permanent night duty; nobody argued, as this meant much less night shift for everyone else.

'Twas the beginning of the end.

One night, a GP came in to attend a woman who was about to deliver. He was a pompous, supercilious arse. The baby was born white and floppy. He took the child to the resuscitation trolley and administered oxygen. When the baby hadn't improved after about two minutes, he decided to intubate (insert a tube into the trachea for the purposes of ventilation). It was clear the child would require oxygen support and probable transfer to another facility.

Now, inserting an intubation tube down a tiny bronchus requires considerable skill. It soon became clear to me that the GP wasn't skilled in neonatal intubation and was way out of his depth. The doctor panicked and sweating, ended up lacerating the larynx and puncturing the trachea. The child was retrieved by the Newborn and Paediatric Emergency Transport Service (NETS), stabilised and airlifted with his mother to Sydney. I understand the little boy survived, but the injuries he sustained would cause him difficulties and complications in the future. I doubt he would have been able to speak properly even with surgical intervention. Again, I question the level of investigation into yet another adverse outcome, as no one asked me for a report. Patterns unchanging...

I worked a night shift that was a game-changer for me and the very last straw. I was caring for a woman who was well advanced in labour. I estimated delivery to be about thirty minutes away. This was the patient's third baby. After about thirty minutes of pushing, there was little progress in the descent of the head. I telephoned the GP and apprised him of the situation. He said he would come to the hospital. About twenty minutes later, he arrived, red-eyed and clearly the worse for wear. The acrid fumes of alcohol filled the room. The husband of the patient looked at me in horror. The woman was also aware that the doctor was drunk.

After another few pushes, it was clear this baby wasn't about to budge. Swaying, he looked at me. "Get me a pair of Wrigley's." (Forceps).

Shit! This was not going to go well. I retrieved the forceps and then quickly set up the resuscitation trolley for the baby. The doctor was clumsy and very clearly rattled as he clanged the forceps blades with shaking hands. After two attempts to insert the blades, I guided his hands and then clicked the handles locked. After what seemed like forever, the baby was born—white and not breathing. As soon as the umbilical cord was cut, I took the child to the resuscitation trolley, placed a mask over his mouth and nose, and hand-bagged him with oxygen, all the while rubbing him with a towel to stimulate him. The silent doctor sat on a metal stool, watching me. I continued to 'bag' the now pink baby when he let out an indignant cry. The doctor turned back to face the patient, delivered the placenta, sutured the episiotomy, offered wooden congratulations and left the building.

You're welcome!

I finished work at 7:30am. I tendered my resignation to Matron at 8am.

5

In 1982, I moved back to Sydney and started work again at my old hospital. I was so glad to be back, supported by highly competent people I knew had my back. Slowly, I started to feel safe again in the workplace. I will always value the experience at this hospital because it made me into the midwife I am today.

In 1983, I met the eldest son of my mom's best friend. We had never crossed paths because by the time my family had moved (again) to the gorgeous NSW south coast, he, at 17, had joined the Royal Australian Navy, and I had gone nursing in the New England. At first sight, we both knew we had found the one person destined to be each other's life partner. We were like salt and pepper shakers; we just fit together.

Life was good. I loved my now, fiancé, and I loved my job.

I had a really good mate, P., who today continues to be a lifelong friend. Like me, she is a midwife who worked at the same Sydney hospital. As is a nurse's lot, too often, events such as needle stick injuries or blood/body fluid splashes to the eyes or mucus membranes result from participating in nursing/midwifery care. The protocol was that blood was to be collected from the nurse and the patient to ensure the nurse has not contracted Hepatitis B. Remember, this was the time of the HIV/AIDS era in Australia. Midwives are particularly at risk due to the amount of blood and body fluids encountered during birthing or antenatal and postnatal haemorrhage. P. and I were chatting when she mentioned receiving a Letter of Demand, a Final Notice for $20.00AU. The itemised cost was for pathology expenses incurred for blood collection following a needle stick injury. I laughed and told her I had received the exact same notice, which, at the time, I thought was an error, so I threw mine in the bin.

Being endlessly curious individuals, we asked around, and sure enough, a raft of our colleagues received the same notification. Some panicked and paid it immediately to avoid the threat of court action. Others like me thought it was a clerical stuff-up and ditched it into the bin. Now, those who know me know I love a good mystery. In the past, I have often been referred to as 'Sherlock'. If I need an answer, I just cannot let it be. I chase explanations to unanswered questions like a rat up a drainpipe.

After doing our homework, P. and I established that staff are not liable for the cost of pathology services if a needle stick or blood splash occurs. This is a workplace responsibility. We then noticed the only contact details on the letter were the name X. X. Debt Collection Agency, a post office box, and a phone number.

Hmmm... Surely, that couldn't be right.

Back in search of answers, we went, and soon learned the legal responsibilities of businesses in the provision of contact information. We learned that a post office box was unacceptable and a legitimate address and phone number were apparently the minimum advertised information required for any registered business. We were more than intrigued.

Now I understand how curiosity killed the cat.

Like two super sleuths on the tail of some great mystery, and after losing rock /paper/scissors, I rang the phone number on the top of the Letter of Demand. We had no clue what to expect.

Oh Jesus! What came next was totally unexpected! A female voice on the other end of the phone confirmed our call was connected to the Finance Department of the hospital where we both worked. Neither of us saw that coming! I terminated the call without uttering a word. This is when I grasped how conspiracy theories evolve.

Do you think we let sleeping dogs lie? Of course not. After a bit more investigating, we gleaned that employee pathology tests in New South Wales public hospitals are paid for out of a defined bucket of money, like Workers' Compensation payments. When our deductions lead to a final conclusion, it was like being hit with a brick. When the Finance Department issued the fraudulent Letters of Demand threatening court action, it was a 'double dip.'

The costs of the tests were already paid out of whatever the kitty is called for work health-related costs.

What other conclusion, could there be?

This is what I mean about being naive. P. and I made an appointment with the then-Director of Nursing to discuss our evidence and conclusions. Two minutes into the meeting, the Director of Nursing raged. It suddenly became obvious that our allegations were not news to her.

She threw us out of the office. Right! Now, we really wanted to know what was going on. P. and I made an appointment with the Director of Finance. From the moment we entered his office, he clearly had an agenda. After inviting us to sit, he stood and leaned across the desk. He addressed us individually by name as he sneered, "This isn't about mommies and babies, girlies. This is big business, and I suggest you back away right now. You have no idea what you have gotten yourselves into." He intimated that the double dip went as high as the New South Wales Premier. Well, shit.

P. and I were completely broadsided. Firstly, because he knew our names and where we worked, and secondly, he confirmed our suspicions in a veiled threat. The Director of Nursing obviously had briefed him in detail about our visit.

For the first time in my life, I experienced the darkness of the unknown and the fear accompanying it. I didn't feel threatened exactly, but I was on higher alert than usual. So was P. Not long after the meeting with the Director of Finance, her house was broken into. Nothing was taken, but things were moved from their usual places—a clear message that someone had been there. That was it—we were officially warned off. Sherlock and Watson hung up their hats and went out of business.

Just before I made my next career move, I experienced my first episode of Superior Ventricular Tachycardia (SVT). This is a cardiac condition that can be brought on by extreme stress, resulting in significant palpitations. I was looking after a woman in labour. She had an acute psychiatric illness and a history of violence. She was abusive and aggressive. She was also very distressed and well-advanced in labour. Suddenly, she stood on the bed, reached up, grabbed the handle of the huge multi-globed spotlight attached to the ceiling and started to swing off it like Tarzan. The light would have weighed a ton, and the risk of her bringing it and the whole ceiling down on top of herself and me was very real. I tried unsuccessfully, to talk her down. I hit the emergency button. Staff came running from everywhere. Still hanging from the light fitting, the woman kicked out at me viciously and caught me square in the face. I was knocked to the ground. A rush of raw fury filled my chest.

The next thing I knew, I woke up in the Resuscitation Room attached to a cardiac monitor. My heart rate was just over 200 beats a minute. My experience of SVT, instead of any previous history, was put down to extreme stress. I was told to go home and I would be right by morning. I had been viciously assaulted. Apparently, that was an expected part of the job.

I don't bloody think so.

Being a midwife is both rewarding and challenging. Birthing is a fantastic experience. To be present to welcome a new family member into the world is, for the most part, a true privilege—but not always. Sometimes, it is just so hard not to be judgemental.

I recall taking over the care of a woman who was a known intravenous drug user whose drug of choice was heroin. She was admitted in established labour with her fifth child; all four previous children were in the care of the State. On admission, it was apparent to me, that she was under the effect of some substance—presumably heroin as there were fresh track marks on her arms. The labour proceeded quickly. Being a high-risk pregnancy, the foetus was monitored continuously. The patient was abusive and struck out at me many times with her fists. It was extremely difficult to keep the baby monitored as the patient was uncooperative. Not long after she was admitted, she started to push. The baby's heartbeat plummeted from between 140 to 150 beats per minute to 100 beats per minute. I tried to get her to stop pushing as I ducked flying fists when she spat, "Fuck off, bitch."

I rang the emergency bell, and the team leader came in, ascertained the situation and urgently paged the Neonatal Registrar. This baby was in trouble. The heart rate slowly decelerated to 40 beats per minute, 30 beats per minute, 20 beats per minute...

As the head had crowned, the baby suffered a cardiac arrest from the combined effects of the recently injected heroin and the additional stress of labour. The little boy was delivered, not breathing, with no heartbeat. The Neonatal Registrars at this hospital were very experienced and expert in high-level resuscitation. The baby was ventilated and given drugs, only to survive as the latest unwanted baby—another victim of having lost in the parent lottery by being born to a woman who could never be trusted to care or provide for him. As the baby was wheeled out of the room and taken to Neonatal Intensive Care, the woman abused everyone present, screaming vitriol that we were incompetent and were responsible for her baby needing Intensive Care.

Some people just have no insight. Enough. In truth, I was done with aggressive, violent patients. I was tired of the disrespect. This nomad had itchy feet. I needed a new job. I applied for a Nurse Manager Level 3 (Supervisor) position for the Delivery Suite in a peripheral Sydney hospital in another Area Health Service. I got the job! This was a brand-new service. The hospital was originally built in 1977 without either a maternity unit or a mortuary — two significant oversights if ever there were any. Local women had been required to go to a nearby hospital offering maternity services since 1902. I guess the deceased likewise went to the same facility.

This job was a marvellous challenge. We opened the doors without staff. Recruitment ended with many of the midwives being brand-new graduates. I often chuckle when I remember that we opened the service without an oxygen nipple to bless ourselves with. This meant that if oxygen was required, there was no means of connecting the oxygen supply to the tubing attached to the patient. The lessons of my old hospital came in very handy. My number one priority was education and in-service, clinical skills registers, orientation to team leading, and so much more. Also, I introduced reference points for the staff in the form of policy and procedure manuals. There was continuity of practice, the staff flourished and became very skilled. I was so proud of them.

I have always been a take-charge kind of girl. I am also a 'fixer,' which is a quality that is often, to my great detriment. I get involved in issues that are not mine to solve. I relish responsibility and am entrepreneurial in my practice. As an out-of-the-box, global thinker, I love nothing more than a complex issue that requires a solution.

Bliss.

I never really understood why I am the way I am, until after my appointment as the manager of the Delivery Suite. All of the hospital's managers were invited to attend a Myers-Briggs conference. The purpose of the conference was to examine different management styles to gain an understanding of why managers behave as they do.

More and more, today's potential leaders are often subjected to psycho-parametric testing as part of the interview process. All participants at the conference undertook the Myers-Briggs Type Indicator assessment. I, it seems, am an ENTJ, which equates to:

E: Extraverted

N: Intuitive

T: Thinking

J: Judging

According to Myers Briggs, personalities can be defined by their character traits. It is estimated that 2-5% of all people are ENTJs, of which less than 1% are women. ENTJs are strategic leaders who are motivated to organise change. They have an innate, built-in radar that addresses inefficiencies and can conceptualise system problem resolution. They are in for the long haul and are focused on long-range plans to accomplish their vision. They excel at logical reasoning (my husband's nickname for me is Spock) and are usually articulate and quick-witted. ENTJs are analytical and objective and like bringing order to the world around them. Reviewing system or process flaws and participating in finding the solution, gives ENTJ great satisfaction. They are assertive and enjoy taking charge (no surprises there); they see their role as leaders and managers, organising people and processes to achieve their goals. Some historical examples of ENTJs are Winston Churchill, Margaret Thatcher, Julius Caesar, Bill Gates and Steve Jobs.

This finding was not a surprise to me but rather, an affirmation of why I am incapable of turning a blind eye to adverse outcomes or poor practice and possess such a strong sense of determination and social justice. This is why it is imperative that I consider advocating for patients not only a part of my role as a nurse but also a mandatory practice. Based on this newfound knowledge, it is hardly surprising that I heeded the call to a position in management.

The experience of being a pupil midwife was burned into my soul. The witness of births where the women were not aware they were being watched, to me, is nothing short of voyeurism. Also, being sent into a room to 'do the delivery', having never met the woman or established any rapport with her, is a tick-box exercise. In midwifery practice, the true learning is in the journey: being with the woman from the onset of labour, observing the physical changes, monitoring the baby and its descent into the pelvis and most importantly, understanding the woman's wishes and birth plan. Having a baby is a momentous, memorable event. As a midwife, I am ethically bound to assist the woman in any way I can to ensure she and the baby are delivered safely.

My previous midwifery experiences have had a profound effect on my leadership style. A midwifery training school was established, and pupil midwives were soon on the wards and working in the Delivery Suite. Blessedly, achieving a midwifery qualification in 1986 was still 100% hospital-based. Today, the education of nurses and midwives is a very different story. Nursing and midwifery theory is gained from university classrooms, which is appropriate as today, successful study as a Midwife, results in a degree qualification. In my view, with inadequate face-to-face interaction with actual patients, clinical learning is problematic and contributes to early attrition of newly graduated nurses and midwives from the profession. Nursing is a hands-on job, and nurses have never worked harder than they do today, caring for patients of acuity that 20 years ago would have seen them cared for in High Dependency Units. The skills required to be a competent nurse/midwife cannot be drawn from nursing theory alone but rather in combination, with participation in patient care. I do not believe nursing education has struck the right partnership with the clinical providers and students, with the registered nurses/midwives of the future — paying the price. Being a new graduate nurse/midwife who arrives at the workplace clinically unprepared to do the job is tough. Sink or swim, or get thrown to the wolves; either way, gaining the skills that should have been garnered while still a student is hard. New graduate registered nurses require mentorship and supervision to acquire the skills necessary to achieve competency in clinical skills. The situation for new graduate midwives is no different.

My priority as the manager of the Delivery Suite was to foster a culture of professional respect for the women and their plans for labour. Many of the original midwives were very inexperienced. It was imperative that they were offered education and support to enable them to accept and provide expected care. The mandatory sign-off of the occasions of attended clinical procedures was achieved by being allocated to the woman from admission to the Delivery Suite until she delivered. If the pupil midwife was not assigned to the woman but required as a 'witness' (witness the birth) or to receive a baby, the pupil was required to introduce him/herself to the patient and her partner and seek their permission to be in the room at the time of the birth. The rights of the patient were observed at all times.

The hospital was soon accredited to accept medical students. Some were allocated to work in the Delivery Suite. Medical students are unqualified medical officers in the very junior stages of their training. I remember one student arriving at the Delivery Suite around 9am. He was a pompous, arrogant, young upstart who wore the obligatory crisp white doctors' coat and a stethoscope around his neck. I intercepted him in the corridor and asked if I could help him. He introduced himself and advised me he was here to deliver a baby! He brushed invisible lint from the front of his coat and then regarded me with contempt.

Hmmm...

I loathe supercilious people who speak down to others. I have a particular dislike for medical officers who possess this character trait. I have worked with medical officers who considered themselves God's gift to humanity. It never ends well. I informed the medical student that the shift changeover was at 7am sharp. As he was two hours late for the morning handover, he had two choices: come back at 2pm for the afternoon handover and stay for the entire shift, which ended at 10:30pm, or return the next day at 7am and join the morning handover. He sneered at me and regarded me as if I were an impaired person. "You don't seem to understand. I am the son of Professor X; therefore, those rules don't apply to me."

I stepped closer to him and spoke in a quiet but deliberate tone, "I don't care if your father is Moses himself. In this Delivery Suite, as a medical student, you are expected to arrive ready for handover at 7am or 2pm. This information was issued to you along with your roster as part of the information package all medical students receive before starting this rotation. After handover, as a medical student, you will be assigned to work with a senior midwife who will mentor and supervise your practice. Oh, and you may not be aware, although I believe it is mentioned in the information package that all the staff here wear scrubs. There are no exceptions; we are a team. You will be expected to change into scrubs like everyone else, and there is no need to wear your stethoscope. There are stethoscopes in each of the suites."

He looked at me as if I had asked him to share a bed with a person with the plague, then scoffed at me, "Pfft. Look, I'm here because I have to be; I couldn't give two shits about you or your rules."

I regarded him for a moment before I spoke. Depending on how I handled this situation there could be major ramifications for me.

Consequences, be damned. I asked him, "Is that your final decision?'

Imperious, he looked down his nose and said, "Yes, it is."

I considered him carefully, imagining the shit-storm that would unfold next, but I didn't care. The women deserved respect, and clearly, if what I had experienced of his attitude was anything to go by, he was not about to respect anyone.

"As you have indicated your unwillingness to accept the routines in place for medical students on rotation to Delivery Suite, I accept your decision. Leave now and don't come back. Your rotation is herewith cancelled. I will advise the Medical

Intake Officer of the events of this morning. Good day to you."

I waited for him to leave. His eyes bugged in disbelief as he turned and walked towards the front door. Shit! Now I had done it!

I confessed my actions to the Divisional Manager, who roared laughing. She took it upon herself to inform the Medical Intake Officer (given that she held greater authority and wielded a bigger stick than I did). I never heard another word about the event. This was a lesson that would serve this young man well in the future. I hope his ego allowed him to realise that.

In 1987, a year after I accepted the Manager of Delivery Suite job, I gave birth to my first child, a son, and yes, Matron was less than impressed that I was on maternity leave within a year of accepting the position. Towards the end of the pregnancy, I became inexplicably fearful for the welfare of my baby. I kept having a terrifying, recurring dream that something was going to go terribly wrong. I tried not to give in to the residual memories. I was fairly certain that all women about to give birth experience worry for their offspring.

My dad and my much-loved father-in-law spent the time I was in labour sitting in the hospital waiting room, watching the Rugby League. Apparently, my timing is terrible, as my baby was born before the full-time whistle. The poppies were all for hanging back for the final whistle after which a, they would make their way into the Delivery Suite, and welcome the first grandchild for both sides of the family. Predictably, the nannas were having none of that. Football be damned! My mother-in-law (God bless her beautiful soul) arranged with the receptionist to switch off the waiting room television. Then the two formidable women, both suffering with a bad case of granny lust ushered the two howling poppies into the Delivery Suite. They couldn't get to my son fast enough.

My boy, 'N.', is one of my life's great joys. At four months of age, the day after his second round of vaccinations, he had a high temperature, which is to be expected. I gave him a dose of Paracetamol, and his temperature settled. As I was on maternity leave, I was doing weekend agency shifts — that way, N. always had one parent with him. On the day of the fever, I worked a morning shift in Neonatal Intensive Care at my old hospital. My husband called me to say something was wrong with N; he was wet with sweat, and he couldn't wake him up. That was when I heard a sound through the phone that no parent ever wants to hear — the sound of a child in acute respiratory distress.

I am usually good in a crisis, but I now understand absolute, off the charts, panic. I left the shift and cannot recall the hour-long trip home. When inside our house, my worst fears were confirmed. N. had a raging fever, and he was having continuous seizures. I picked him up and just walked and walked and walked around the house with him in my arms, talking to him, saying over and over, 'Don't you die, please don't you die.' The adrenaline kicked the ENTJ into action, and I entered nurse mode. I called the ambulance, and N. was transported to the hospital, where I was the manager of the Delivery Suite. A paediatrician whom often attended Delivery Suite and whom I had great respect for had been contacted. He was on hand when the ambulance arrived. I remember being in the Acute Area of the Emergency Department on autopilot, doing the things that I would do if any other child had been likewise admitted. The staff felt for me and gently reminded me that my role today was mother, not nurse. I returned to the waiting room, feeling more helpless than I have ever felt before. My husband and I paced the corridors, waiting for answers.

I will never forget the paediatrician's solemn expression as he walked out of the Acute Area. He looked me straight in the eye, pain etched into his face. "Kath, I'm so sorry; N. has had a massive cerebral haemorrhage. He's going to die."

The world stopped. The paediatrician arranged for my son to be transferred to a major Sydney Paediatric hospital. He put his arm around me and said, "This," and gestured at the waiting ambulance, "it won't make any difference to the outcome, but you will know everything that could have been done will have been done. I am so sorry."

N. was in Intensive Care and continued to have continuous seizures despite massive doses of anticonvulsants. The doctors painted a very bleak picture. Eventually, after two of the longest days in my life, the drugs won and the seizures stopped. N. was downgraded to the paediatric neurological ward. My tiny boy had suffered a massive stroke. We could not have imagined the challenges to come, in the rearing of a brain-injured child.

Thank God for family. My folks and my husband's folks and siblings, as well as our friends, were constant in their support for us. I couldn't begin to imagine what it would be like to go through this terrible time without them. I stayed on the ward with N. and slept in the parent's room - a narrow single room with an ensuite. One night, N. was in his cot on the ward, was distressed and crying, and nothing I did settled him. I admit I was sleep-deprived, reactive and cranky. That was when I noticed a child of maybe three years of age lying on the floor at the feet of a nurse sitting at the nurses' station. I lifted N. out of his cot and walked towards her. Her eyes bugged at my unmistakable look of horror. She flapped her hand over the little body on the linoleum, as she rapid fired, "Oh, this is S. He fits continuously. We keep him here with us to keep an eye on him."

It took every bit of restraint not to slap her.

As I had witnessed substandard care by this nurse, I informed her I was taking N. to the parent's room to sleep with me. She became most indignant. "No, that is against hospital policy. Your son needs close observation! I will contact the After-Hours Manager and Security."

I am not a person to be tangled with at the best of times, but when it comes to my precious offspring, I am a she-bear. I regarded the nurse with absolute contempt and dipped my head towards S., who was still convulsing on the floor.

"You call this close observation? Just so as you know, I'm a Registered Nurse too! And I can assure you I have a bloody sight more experience than you do. Call whomever you like. Call the fucking Prime Minister for all I care. My son and I are going to bed, and if you know what's good for you, you will leave his care to me."

I took my boy to bed, breastfed him, and he had the first good night's sleep since we had left home. The nurses brought his medications to him when they were due, then left us in peace, and that is how it was until we were discharged home. N. experienced a residual complete left-sided weakness, which has persisted to this day. But I am my father's daughter. I did whatever it took to help my son to recover and grow to be the best person he could be. My husband and I pushed him endlessly with physical therapy. I am 100% responsible for the fact that, as a child, he didn't sleep through the night until he was seven years of age. I would hover over him constantly, to make sure he was breathing. My constant hovering interruptions disrupted his sleep cycles. Anyone who has lived with a brain-injured person will know that irrational behaviour and anger and violence are a part of everyday life. We pushed him even harder with anger management strategies. Today, he is as sharp as a tack, with five children of his own. He still has residual clonic movements in his left hand, but so what? He survived. He is an intelligent, loving human being whom we adore. The world is a better place for having him in it.

People who know N.'s history, often say, "Oh, so you're one of those who are anti-immunisation?"

My answer to that is simple. "No, I am not against immunisation. In a responsible society, we must do what is for the greater good, and immunisation is for the greater good."

In 1988, a few months after N. had been discharged from hospital, we travelled 700kms to spend two weeks with my Mom and Dad who had finally stopped moving around and had put down roots. They literally built their house with their own hands. The local community rallied as Dad's family had been locals for years. Finally, they committed to settling down and their first house became a home. They named the house Dunmovin and had the name engraved on a plaque which Dad nailed with pride near the front door.

Dad was one of thirteen children. His family had lived about 40 miles from the closest village. Back then, there were precious few mod cons — no electricity, no telephones and no television, only kerosene lamps and a gas refrigerator. He taught me how to be a principled human being and about social justice. The bush was his home and he knew it like the back of his hand. He taught me which tree gave the best wood to cook the Sunday roast and which ones would fill the house with smoke. His sense of humour never ceased to make me laugh and he had a saying for every occasion. He would say things like 'I'll tell ya somethin', that bloke is about as useful as a screen door on a submarine.' He was a hoot and an all-round great man. Dad was the one who taught me to MacGyver — that is, to make do with what was available and use common sense to solve problems. He used to say never throw anything away, 'cause it's bound to come in handy and only after seven years should I even think about disposing of things into the bin.

He used to regale us with the story of the time when he and his siblings all caught whooping cough. Grandma treated them with a special mixture, only known to her, that contained the juice of prickly pear. She was a Shaman of sorts. Apparently prickly pear has a high laxative effect which resulted, according to Dad, in poopin' while whoopin'. She also made this amazing ointment that would cure chronic leg ulcers. People from all over Australia who knew of it, would contact her for a tin of her secret remedy. Perhaps her greatest act of spite towards me was that she took all her secrets to the grave and didn't share her recipes or her knowledge with me.

My parents were always great role models — family first, family always. They adored N. and he was my Dad's pride and joy. I fondly remember when we visited how he used to sit him on his lap while watching television, talking to him and calling him his 'little mate'. I also remember the day when it was time to return home, Dad's voice was uncharacteristically earnest when he said to me, "You make sure you look after this boy." I swear his eyes were moist. I was confused.

On the 1st of August 1988, my world spun off its axis when my larger-than-life Dad passed away most unexpectedly. He was aged just 56 and was one of the most brilliant people I have ever had the privilege to know. He was illiterate which presented many challenges for him during his life. His illiteracy was the reason he instilled the importance of education in me. My Mom was just 49 years old and suddenly, she was a widow. Dunmovin' was right. Fuck!

Mom and Dad had lived a very stereotypical type of life, Dad was the bread winner and Mom was the homemaker. She didn't drive and had been married to the love of her life since she was 17 years of age. Now she was all alone and life was very confronting for her. She didn't drive, she didn't chop wood and she didn't pour concrete for garden beds. Today she has mastered all of those skills. She works harder than anyone I know and I am so proud of her. The day after Dad passed, she said to me, frowning, "I don't understand why the rest of the world hasn't stopped, mine has."

She grieved as she became independent. She taught me to never give up and that anything is possible if you put your mind and your back into it. I love her dearly. I was 30 years old when I endured that dreadful year of firsts — first Christmas without him,

9th January — his birthday without him, Mom's birthday without him, the first Easter without him, N.'s first birthday without him.

Finally, the calendar ticked over to 1989. That somehow made life a little easier. I grieved for my Dad for a very long time, I still do, but I cherish the lessons he taught me about 'doing the right thing' and the importance of education and family. I know he watches over me. I also know that if I am getting a bit too big for my britches, he finds a way of giving me the message to tell me to pull my head in. I love you Dad, I always have and I always will. Your ideals are my ideals, and I am very glad of it.

Somehow, life went on. Nursing as a profession offers great satisfaction but it pays a pittance. It seems professional status with blue collar wages is good enough for nurses. But the wolf was clawing at the door. I needed to go back to work. As I was still on maternity leave, my husband cared for N. (hovered like a hawk) while I continued to pick up weekend shifts working with the nursing agency. I experienced highly confronting situations like trying to cajole a sedated but screaming child who was submerged in a warm bath with Lux Flakes (pure soap) to soak the serous exudate from her horrendously burned body. Having been through the experience with N. each one of her screams was like a knife in my heart. I vowed never to accept a shift in a Paediatric ward again. I digress. In my lifetime, whenever I say never, it is guaranteed I will do whatever I was never going to do

– again. I had nightmares about that poor child for months. I still think about her.

I recall the day I was booked for a day shift on an adult Neurology ward in a major teaching hospital where I met one of Australia's most famous women's magazine columnists. She had undergone brain surgery to remove a tumour. The top of her skull had yet to be replaced to allow for reduction of the swelling and for healing. She wore her head bandages covered by a silk scarf with aplomb. She was just so quick witted, and her lips were always stylishly painted in a vivid shade of red lippie. I liked her immediately. She shared some great gossip with me.

On that same day, I encountered an early forty-something man whom I had been informed had been a highly successful businessman with a lovely wife and children. He had stopped to change a flat tyre late in the evening while driving home along a Sydney freeway and was struck by another car. He incurred horrendous head injuries that left him a vacant shell who didn't recognise his family. He would walk around aimlessly as if so terribly lost. He had an alarm bracelet on his wrist to alert staff when he invariably tried to wander out of the ward, which happened at least fifty times a day and also at night. It is a terrible thing to say, but it would have been kinder to the patient and his family if he had died outright of his injuries. They would have grieved for him, and he would have been at peace. In the short time I spent with this man, just once, I am certain I saw the glimmer of cognisance; for an instant he seemed to remember who he was and what had happened, then it was all gone again behind those vacant blue eyes, into the depths of his damaged brain. I prayed that I was wrong. That would just have been too cruel. I have never forgotten him.

I returned from maternity leave exhausted, but very much in love with my son.

The medical staff found my type of leadership and commitment to the development of a team of midwives who could practice autonomously to be a far cry from midwifery practice they had become accustomed to at the nearby hospital. There the medical model was alive and well and if the obstetrician told the midwife to jump, he or she would ask how high and never question what was asked of them. Not so with my team. From the first day we opened our doors, the midwives were encouraged to think scientifically and to question (God forbid!) if they thought a patient might come to harm.

Over the years, the medical staff and I had a good many discussions that usually started with "Well, the way we have always done things has been good enough, why do we need to change?" Slowly they all came around and we were a good team. However, there was one anaesthetist that I never won over, no matter how hard I argued for change. All of the midwives were taught to 'top up' epidurals. That means when an epidural had been inserted, the drug that masks the pain over time wears off and the drug needs to be topped up' to ensure the epidural continues to be functional. I had attended this procedure many times at my old hospital and was accredited as being competent to do so. All of the Delivery Suite midwives received the same education and were accredited via a clinical competency register. However, this particular anaesthetist — a crusty old bugger if there ever was one — was famous for his gruff manner and his absolute lack of tact. He would come to Delivery Suite when paged to insert an epidural. If the woman was overweight, he would say without fail, "If you don't lose weight you're going to die."

He was of the view that midwives were not competent to top up epidurals. This was despite the fact he had reviewed and signed off on the education, lecture information and the clinical assessment routine. However, if a woman was labouring in the wee hours of the morning and required a top up between the hours of 10pm and 7am, he had a standing order that the on-duty resident, who had never done an anaesthetics term, let alone topped up an epidural, was to be called and the senior midwife on duty was to supervise the procedure and guide the resident where necessary. Only when convenient and advantageous to him did he recognise the abilities of the midwives.

Over time and through a sequence of events, I acquired a reputation for being a strong patient advocate. One such time was when a local VIP gave birth in the Delivery Suite in the early hours of the morning. Just before lunch, I received a directive from the Divisional Leader of Maternity Services that a local MP had contacted the Director of Nursing for details such as the time of birth, sex and the weight of the baby. Seriously? I advised the Divisional Leader to inform the MP that he should buy flowers, visit the woman and allow her to share her good news. The Director of Nursing was flabbergasted that I refused to provide the information, despite being directed to do so. I would not budge on the issue. Patient confidentiality is not a privilege, it is the right of every patient in our care. It is also a tenet of responsibility for professional nurses. I later found out this particular MP was a powerful, influential who was not used to being told no. Not on my watch.

There are some people that cross your path in life that you never forget. One of those people was a midwife who came to work with me. She was energetic, very experienced and a damn fine clinician. 'E.' was loud and had a penchant for swearing. She was the type of person that called a spade a 'fucking shovel'. I admired her skills, and I liked her a lot. Like me, she was a strong patient advocate who would stand her ground against any medical officer if she believed the patient was risk of harm.

There were two particular events involving E. that will stay for me for eternity. One afternoon shift, she was caring for a woman who was labouring with a stillborn full-term infant. The death of a baby whether it be just post-conception or at full-term is a tragedy. Everyone in the room was understandably extremely upset — even E., a seriously hard arsed midwife — shed tears of grief for this poor family. As the labour progressed it became clear that the woman would soon deliver her dead child. The husband of the woman asked E. if she would offer a blessing for the child when it was born. He explained that his clergy would not offer a sacrament as the child was no longer alive and therefore in his view, there was no soul left to pray for. E. explained to me what the husband had requested. I was dumbfounded that any person of the church could be so judgemental and heartless in the face of such grief and pain.

I agreed that we should try to meet the parents' wishes. As Christians, a blessing for their child would give them comfort in their time of absolute need. I am of the Salvation Army faith, so I am well practiced in helping others, prayers and Christian beliefs. I rummaged around and found a pretty glass dish and filled the container with warm water — I don't know why, but cold water in some way seemed wrong. Together, E. and I went back into the Delivery Suite. The woman was very distressed and the urge to push had started. We all sat quietly around the bed and cried for the lost life and for the journey of grief that awaited these two people. Blessedly, the baby was born quickly. She was perfect, with no obvious sign of the cause of her demise. She was white with blue lips and closed eyes. E. sobbed as she wrapped the tiny body in a bunny rug and handed her to her mother.

God it was heartbreaking. I am crying again as I write this.

It was then that E. reached for the little glass container, dipped her fingers in the water and started to make the sign of the cross on the baby's forehead. "In the name of the Father and the Son and the…" There was a long pause and she looked at me with eyes like a rabbit stunned by oncoming headlights. "Oh fuck! There's three of them! I know there's another one!"

I blurted "And the Holy Ghost, Amen."

There was deadly silence when suddenly the parents burst out laughing. E. hugged them both as she cried and said, "I am so sorry! I was never much for church!"

Not long after the birth, distressed family members started to arrive. As a family, they spent quiet time with the baby until the parents sadly were ready to part with her. They opted to go home directly from Delivery Suite rather than be transferred to the Postnatal Ward, where there were ecstatic new mothers and crying babies. As they were leaving, the woman handed me a pretty, hand crocheted lacy bunny rug and lovely embroidered baby clothes. She couldn't speak; her tears stole her voice. Her husband said, "We want Mary-Rose buried in these clothes. Can you make sure that someone dresses her for her burial?"

Tears ran down my face as I assured them, I would personally ensure the baby was dressed in her beautiful clothes to make her final journey.

Being a midwife brings great joy and great sorrow. It also brings the unexpected. As fate would have it, a couple of days later, I received a call from the couple whose baby had died. E. also happened to be on duty. A few hours earlier, I had been notified by the mortuary attendant that the baby's body was to be collected around lunch time and that the parents had requested to have a final viewing. E. offered to go to the mortuary and dress Mary-Rose (the baby) for her parents, to enable them to say their goodbyes and have one last hold of her mortal body.

After about an hour, the phone rang, it was E. She was frantic. "Kath! There's a fucking problem!"

I was perplexed. "What do you mean there is a problem? Have the parents arrived? Is everything okay?"

"No thank Christ they haven't arrived yet! The bloody fridge is playing up! Mary-Rose is frozen! As in, ice cube, frozen!"

All I could envisage was the parents arriving to find their beloved child frozen like and anatomical specimen.

E. was nearly hysterical. "It gets fucking worse. As I dressed Mary-Rose, something snapped — you know — fucking frozen, snapped! I think it was the shoulder because nothing has fallen off!"

The ENTJ in me, in response to the visual scene in my brain, launched into action. "Continue to dress the baby. For Christ's sake just be careful to not snap off anything else. Wrap the baby tightly in the shawl and pray to God that the parents don't want her unwrapped. Explain to them that rigor mortis makes the body very stiff and the baby is so cold because refrigeration is required to preserve the body until the time of the burial." The parents came and sat in the viewing room and held little Mary-Rose and said their goodbyes. Amen to that.

Years later E. attended the birth of a baby whose shoulders were too big to pass through the birth canal. This is called shoulder dystocia and it is an obstetric emergency. There are only two options; either try to rotate the shoulders so that they align in the correct position, which is vertical with the pubic bone, or apply extreme downward traction to free the first shoulder blade out from under the pubic bone, then the second. This is a very dangerous manoeuvre for the baby, as the collar bones and shoulder blades are at significant risk of fracture. The ultimate complication is that the shoulders are just too big and that the baby cannot be delivered vaginally. At this stage of delivery, caesarean section is not an option for the head is delivered and the body is too far down into the birth canal. E. conducted a most complicated delivery, determined to deliver this baby alive. She gave it everything she had and was left in a lather of sweat. She was in pain, shaky and exhausted. She had pushed past her own pain barrier and had incurred a full thickness tear of the rotator cuff in her shoulder. Thanks to her, the baby was born, resuscitated and recovered. She never again worked as a Delivery Suite midwife due to chronic pain and lack of strength in her shoulder. The profession of midwifery is poorer today for the loss of her skills.

In 1990, ten years had passed since the transfer of nurse education to the tertiary sector. There was a growing nervousness among the 'hospital trained' midwives that their qualifications might be somehow regarded as inferior. It makes me furious to hear that, nurses who trained in the hospital system went to university to undertake the Bachelor of Health Science, Nursing; a qualification they already held, as if to legitimise the original qualification. So much for solidarity and value for the excellent training we received. It is amusing when you think about it, given that we Baby Boomers are the role models, mentors and supervisors for new graduate registered nurses. We were the ones who taught them their clinical skills.

In 1991, I was 33 years old when I gave birth to my second child — a little girl who is another great blessing in my life. She is very similar me in that she has a strong sense of social justice and like me, she is a warrior. However, blessedly she does not have my heart of glass. Life's crap slides off her like she is made of Teflon.

I am so very glad. She and her brother are decent human beings whom I will always consider to be my greatest achievements.

One of the midwives I worked with and I were great mates. We decided it would be a good idea if we both enrolled in a Bachelor of Health Management at the University of New England. Our study plan was to be external students. Our candidature was accepted and we were welcomed into the world of academic study. What a hoot. As external study students, we were required to attend residential schools that were a week in duration, twice per year of enrolment. Those were great days! We had lots of laughs with me and my trusty breast pump expressing milk so that I wouldn't explode until I got back to my gorgeous little girl, whose pre-pumped and frozen sustenance was safely stored in our freezer — a supply any dairy farmer would have been proud of.

It was during these residential schools that I met (then) Dr Jeanne Madison, who introduced me to Quality Management and how health organisations grow and prosper while developing the most important resource — the people who do the job. I also met Professor Victor Minichiello, who taught me, through qualitative research, how to see the world through the eyes of others. Meeting these two extremely talented people ignited a spark in me and a love for qualitative research and academic study. Both of these people would later be very influential in my life. I felt like I had come home... Then Fate played another hand....

I was approached by management to ask if I was interested in relieving in the role of an After-Hours Senior Nurse Manager - Level 2. This is the person who is the caretaker of the hospital outside of business hours. During this time, I became acquainted with three women who, like me, took their nursing responsibilities very seriously. They would later play a big part in my future.

Back in those days, nurses could chop and change roles without the position being advertised or interviews held. That just would not happen today. As an After-Hours Manager, I was required to visit each of the clinical areas of the hospital. I came to know a lot of the staff. The first two were Meadhbh who was wonderfully Irish, and Yanaha, who were both Clinical Nurse Specialists in operating theatre. They were very skilled clinicians and professional nurses whom I held great respect for. Later that year, a young woman named Narissa who joined the After-Hours Senior Nurse Managers. She was vivacious, wilful and determined. She had strong opinions about most things. By nature, she was volatile, and I trod carefully around her.

Corruption, I have decided, is a nebulous thing. What seems like corrupt behaviour to some, may simply just be a different way of doing things to others. I recall a medical officer in his early thirties who was employed to work in the Emergency Department.

He was likeable, energetic and incredibly knowledgeable for someone at such an early stage in his career. He was like a whirlwind. He would see patients and have them out the door in no time. The nurses loved him because he could clear the waiting room faster than a sailor's fart.

I recall one morning walking down to the Emergency Department when I saw a patient leaning against a wall holding a tea towel wrapped hand against his chest. I smiled as I passed when I heard the doctor say, "Roy how many times have I told you to put the guard on the mill blade? Mate, one of these days you're going to cut your bloody hand off or worse, bleed to death out at the mill."

My internal radar klaxon started blaring. I stopped and turned, pretending to search for something in my folder. The doctor said, "Come on in. Let's see what bloody damage you've done this time. You had a tetanus shot in the surgery when you dropped the axe on your foot, didn't you?"

The patient nodded and followed behind the doctor. Just before they entered the clinical area, the doctor said "I'll fix you up for now and give you a shot of antibiotics. But no more work today, okay? Now today is Tuesday, come to the rooms and see me on Friday. The wound will need to be redressed and I might need to prescribe some more antibiotics."

They both entered the clinical area and the doors closed, leaving me out in the corridor. I couldn't believe it. No wonder the doctor seemed so experienced and had such a well-developed bedside manner. He was a General Practitioner with his own rooms and patients. To work in an Emergency Department and advise patients to return to see him in his rooms made him very popular with the patients that he saw, because he was obviously very caring to arrange that they didn't have to come back to the hospital and sit and wait for God knows how long to be seen. This was also an excellent way to increase his client base and establish his reputation as a wonderful, caring GP. Unfortunately, medical officers are not lawfully entitled to solicit patients in such a fashion. Ethically, but reluctantly, I was bound to report this finding. Personally, I thought he was a good man and a good doctor. But regardless of the face it wears, corruption is corruption.

My experience all those years ago as a third year in the Secondment hospital Emergency Department, left me with a sense of anxiousness and displacement from my comfort zone. I will never forget so many of the things I witnessed there. For example, I was working a day shift and was walking towards the Emergency Department when an ambulance trolley and two ambulance officers came into view. On the trolley was a woman laying on her belly with a bread knife sticking out of the middle of her back. Apparently, the rule of thumb with embedded bread knives is that it is best to leave the offending object in place until the patient is in operating theatres in a controlled situation. I can never look at a bread knife the same way ever again.

I have witnessed brutality. A woman presented to the Emergency Department with mastitis and an extremely painful breast abscess. Instead of admitting the patient to a ward and administering intravenous antibiotics, the medical officer sat the woman on a chair, exposed her breast and stabbed a scalpel, deep into the centre of the abscess. He then grasped her breast and squeezed for all he was worth. Pus squirted everywhere, including all over the woman's trousers. She screamed and screamed. Her face was the colour of chalk. Shocked, I stepped forward as I was sure she was going to faint and slide off the chair. She didn't. She sat there shaking and crying while the medical officer just shook his head and said, "Surely it can't be that bad!"

I spoke to the medical officer after the poor woman had been discharged with a prescription for oral antibiotics. He didn't accept he had done anything wrong. I wrote an incident report and never received a reply.

After that experience I was always anxious when this particular medical officer was on shift. He only ever worked night shift in the Emergency Department. One night, a very dehydrated child was brought into hospital after 24 hours of vomiting and diarrhoea. As is the way with children and dehydration, little people are often difficult to cannulate to administer intravenous fluids. The child was screaming and the mother was screaming. I came to see what all the noise was about and noted at least 10 stab wounds where the medical officer had tried, unsuccessfully, to insert a cannula I said to him, "That's enough, I'll page the Paediatrician on-call to come in."

I left the area to make the phone call when I heard another blood curdling scream. The medical officer had used the intraosseous technique whereby a huge needle is inserted directly into the bone marrow of the child's leg. Intravenous fluids had been commenced. The child and his mother were screaming the place down. Bastard.

Once again, I wrote the obligatory incident report, for which I did not receive any response.

It was time for me to move on. In 1997, I enrolled in the Master of Health Management (hons) at the University of New England. My study subject and thesis was: How do the perceptions and expectations of 4 university prepared Australian new graduate nurses compare with the reality of practising as registered nurse clinicians in the first year of practice? I then did something I swore I would never do. I applied for an After-Hours Manager - Level 3 position at a tertiary hospital not far from the peripheral hospital. The hospital had a terrible reputation. Big mistake. Once again, I should have listened to my gut.

I have worked in some toxic organisations in my career, but nothing on the scale of this place; Bitchy behaviour, arguments, professional jealousy, violence, you name it. This was the place where I witnessed an Emergency Department triage registered nurse lean over the glass screen and tell a patient to "Shut the fuck up."

I pulled her aside to counsel her on her actions. She informed me she had had a shitty shift and that I should just get over myself and that most of these people in the waiting room were pigs anyway! I spoke to her manager the day after. She just laughed at me and said, "Oh you'll get used to her soon enough!"

In the course of my rounds, I met another nurse who would later be influential in my career. Monique was a dynamic Intensive Care Nurse whom I admired. The patient came first, last and always with her. It was our common views on patient advocacy that got us talking in the first place.

After gaining the approval of the Ethics Committee, I recruited new graduates for my master's degree research from the hospital where I worked. I interviewed them three times each over many months. As this was qualitative research, I undertook taped interviews.

One day shift as the After-Hours Manager, I received a call from one of my participants who was also working the morning shift. She was distressed and crying. She stated the Team Leader on shift had just come out of the toilet, was slurred in her speech and was unsteady on her feet. She stated she was certain the Team Leader was stealing narcotics intended for patients and injecting them into herself. I went to the ward and located my participant. She took me to a patient's bedside and showed me the medication chart which indicated the patient had received a narcotic injection thirty minutes prior. The patient was distressed with pain. It was then that the nurse confessed the Team Leader had advised her she didn't need to stay at the bedside and witness the injection (as is protocol). I located the Team Leader and took her into the office. She was clearly affected by some substance. At first, she was angry and didn't want to discuss the issue further. I advised that she could not finish the shift and that a taxi would be provided to take her home. She knew I was obligated to report the incident. We talked about the future and that the (then) Nurses and Midwives Board would make recommendations. She cried, but admitted she needed help. I rang the Pain Service for a name and a contact number in case she was willing to consider rehabilitation.

This event caused the participant in my study to completely decompensate, disillusioned that a nurse could behave so improperly. I counselled her and advised her Nursing Unit Manager of the events so she could support the nurse. My participant could never come to terms with what had happened; she was beyond disillusioned. Her resignation was received a fortnight later. Her lifelong dream to become a registered nurse was over and she was lost to the profession of nursing forever.

When I first came to this 800-bed hospital, there was only ever one After-Hours Senior Nurse Manager on duty. We managed the evening, night and weekend shifts. To say this was a stressful job is an understatement. This role came with a high level of responsibility and accountability. The After-Hours Senior Nurse Manager allocated beds to all patients admitted to the facility, sick leave was replaced, medications retrieved from the Pharmacy, conflict and complaints were addressed and emergency situations such as cardiac arrests were attended. Part of this role was to report sentinel events, also adverse events and outcomes to the Executive team member on call.

There was another Senior Nurse Manager who had worked at this hospital for years. She was aggressive, rude and employed ritual humiliation of staff in public places. At least one of Director of Nursing's children was her godchild, so nepotism was alive and well. She took an instant dislike to me and the feeling was mutual. When I started the job, I advised of the date that my farewell from the previous hospital was to be held and that I could not work on that day. I offered to take a day of annual leave or a rostered day off. As the newbie, this advice was not considered and I was rostered on to a shift. I brought this to the attention of the other Senior Nurse Managers, however there was no negotiation or change made to the roster. I rang in sick on the day of the farewell and attended the function. When I got back from days off, I was summoned to the General Manager's office. When I entered his office, I noted that the Director of Nursing was also seated. It didn't take long before my suspicions were confirmed. He stated that the Senior Nurse Manager had informed him that I had taken a day of sick leave when in fact I attended a night out with my colleagues. This action in his view was fraud and I was going to be held accountable. I explained how the situation had come about and the lengths I had gone to, to ensure the shift would be covered. I also discussed the aggressive unprofessional behaviour of the Senior Nurse Manager towards me and that I was happy to convert the sick leave to annual leave or a rostered day off. He was furious to have been implicated in a bully girl game. The Director of Nursing was told in no uncertain terms to "deal with it!"

I was beginning to realise how this place had earned its reputation.

Sometime later, at the end of a night shift, I received a call from the Team Leader on shift for the Mental Health Unit. There was a scheduled (involuntarily admitted), young First Nations woman who was classified as a Category 1. This meant the patient must be within arm's reach of the staff member assigned to maintain strict surveillance. Regular documented entries and observations were part of the protocol. The woman, in her mid-twenties had a history of frequent admissions for schizophrenia. She was also dead—rigor mortis dead.

As I looked at the body, it was clear had she had been dead for hours. Did the nurse go to sleep and not observe the patient? On questioning her about the preceding hours, she stated, "I noticed the patient had cold feet at around 5.30am, so I rubbed her feet with cream."

Fuck! A First Nations woman, who had been involuntarily scheduled to a psychiatric facility, had died in custody. I notified the Executive team member on call who notified the police and the relatives were informed. This event broke something in me. I think the culmination of my nursing experiences to date, combined with the extreme stress that went with this job, robbed me of my love and respect for nursing, and for nurses. The Coroner's report cited probable cause of death was from an adverse reaction to a medication she was prescribed. The medication in question is known to produce a dose-related prolongation of the QTc interval (a measure of the time between the start of the Q wave and the end of the T wave in the heart's electrical cycle), which is associated with the ability to cause torsades de pointes type arrhythmias, a potentially fatal ventricular tachycardia and sudden death. Again, I question the level of investigation into this death. I wrote my report but was never interviewed by the police. Months later, the woman's relatives contacted me. They were unaccepting of the Coroner's findings. So was I, especially when soon after this event

I encountered the nurse who had been assigned to this patient still working on night shift.

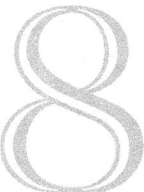

There were some horrible people employed at this hospital — you know the type, those who get their kicks out of persecuting or terrifying others? I remember there was this happy Portuguese man who was employed as a cleaner. One night, he was found in a hysterical state by another staff member. It seems his workmates thought it would be hilarious to fashion the shape of a dead body out of linen and leave it on a trolley parked in a basement corridor for him to find. The poor cleaner was a strict Catholic with a morbid fear of death. He had a significant period of leave because of the impact this event had on him. He did eventually return to the workplace, but he didn't last. He couldn't get past what those men had done to him.

I was starting to feel as though something big was coming, like the lull before a storm. I had no clue as to what...but it was coming. Really shitty events just kept happening. I was starting to agree, I felt jinxed.

One night shift, I received an urgent page from the Mental Health Unit. Crap! When I got there, a young man was standing in the centre of the communal lounge area. He held a long metal pole grasped tight in his hands (it looked like a curtain track fitting). About every thirty seconds or so, he forcibly attempted to jam the rod into one of the many accessible downlight fittings, presumably, to electrocute himself. There were three police officers in attendance. The staff tried to talk the man into surrendering the pole, but he was having none of it. Of great concern to me, was the young male staff member who sat on a lounge chair within easy striking distance of the 'armed' patient, speaking softly, trying to coax him into surrendering the weapon. Suddenly, a police officer grabbed his Capsicum spray canister from his belt and pressed the spray nozzle. I had never experienced Capsicum spray before, and I never want to again. It is truly terrible stuff. It burns the eyes, nose and airways. Also, because it is an aerosol, the spray gets sucked up and circulated by the air conditioning unit and spread throughout, within the range of the unit—which in this case was to the Aged Care Unit! Jesus, Mary Mother of God. Why does this stuff aways happen to me? Fuck!

Twenty aged-care patients and staff, all with streaming eyes and noses had to be evacuated and relocated for the rest of the night, until the on-call maintenance person gave the 'all clear' for patients to be returned to the Aged Care Unit. I was seriously considering getting another job. Again, why do I never listen to what my gut is telling me?

In truth, I wanted to be out of the that hospital, more than anything, but until I could secure another job, I was stuck. This was a fulltime job with a good-sized pay cheque. It seems those two factors anaesthetised my ever-present concerns about this organisation.

I was becoming a different person. I was an automaton from the time I got ready for work until I got home. My shields were up in a pathetic attempt to protect myself from the ever-present assault of poor patient care and adverse outcomes.

One evening shift, I got a 'come now' page from the Emergency Department. As I approached the area, I felt like I had hit a wall. It was very hard to breathe. In the Trauma Room a man had been brought in by ambulance. He was dead. Immediately, the medical officer in charge recognised the smell as the reek of likely ingested organophosphates. When the Hazmat team (an organised group of professionals who are specially trained to handle hazardous materials or dangerous goods) arrived in protective suits like astronauts, complete with breathing apparatus like Darth Vader, I knew we were in trouble. The deceased, apparently consumed the whole 100 tablets in the bottle; one tablet would be enough to kill him. Ingested organophosphates cause the release of toxic fumes from the body. When the Emergency Department staff members started dropping like flies and becoming unwell, it was clear that we had an even bigger problem. This was when it was discovered that the emergency shut off valve in the Trauma

Room could not be activated. This failsafe device was designed to prevent airborne toxins (as in the Capsicum spray and now the organophosphate incident), from being sucked up by the air-conditioning system. The poisonous fumes were circulated into the acute area of the department, which was already full. As luck would have it, the Executive team member on call hadn't left for the day. He came to the department, took charge and did his best to coordinate and control the incident.

The deceased man was so toxic he was placed in a bright orange biochemical holding vat. The lid was permanently sealed, and he was buried that way due to the confirmed organophosphate contamination and the risk the body posed to others. The man was Middle Eastern. His family were bereft that they could not view his body or touch him. The container was under strict Hazmat surveillance and no one was permitted anywhere near it. He was disposed of as biohazardous material. Jesus!

The journalists arrived in droves like hungry wolves to a fresh kill. They took advantage of all of the confusion. It was media heaven. The night sky lit up with flashes from photos being taken of the evacuation of the walking wounded out of the Emergency Department and out into the fresh air. There was no hope of keeping the paparazzi out of the building. However, it was the Hazmat team and the macabre bright orange vat that was the focus of their interest - predators to the end, relishing the last scraps of distress and drama. My husband was watching the late-night television news when he saw me interacting with a person at the front of the hospital, denying access to the building. He guessed I would be late home. He was right.

Just when I thought I had seen just about everything that nursing could throw at me, I was bombarded with a barrage of very stressful events.

One night shift, I received a call from the Team Leader in the Emergency Department who was normally a gregarious, very competent nurse.

"Kath, I think you had better come and have a look at this."

When I asked her what the issue was about, she said she would rather not discuss it on the phone. I went to the department and found the Team Leader with a red Schedule 8 drug register under her arm. These books were used to account for dispensing drugs of addiction. It is a requirement that two clinicians (one of whom must be a registered nurse) check the drug out of the cupboard and witness the administration to the patient. Two signatures are required in the register for every entry. She opened the book to the Pethidine section. I immediately saw why she had called me. There were numerous entries with the same signatures, all of which appeared to have been made with the same pen and with the same hand. The Team Leader then took me to the bed area of a very elderly man, who had been admitted after a fall at home. He was sitting up in bed, head bandaged, enjoying a sandwich and a cup of tea. His medication chart indicated he had received 100mg of Pethidine thirty minutes prior, which clearly wasn't the case. If the gentleman had received that dose of the drug, he would have been very drowsy, if not asleep.

I reviewed the register and it was clear this falsification of drugs administration had been going on for months. The Team Leader advised me who had been responsible for writing up the doses on this shift. I noted the male registered nurse still had the Schedule 8 keys around his neck. I notified the Executive team member on call, who notified the police Drug Squad. When the officers entered the department, the male registered nurse walked out the exit door. The Team Leader and I watched him as he crossed the road over to an adjacent park. When he returned, one police officer took him into a room and performed a strip search while another officer went to the park to search for evidence. The registered nurse was suspended from duty, pending an Inquiry. Six months later, he was found dead in his flat.

By this stage, I was beyond affected by the events at this hospital. I no longer felt safe at work. I was no longer proud to be a nurse and I realised my feelings for the profession of nursing had significantly changed. I have never been a combat soldier, but I can imagine the fear and loathing that each day brings when the assaults just keep occurring. Such was the next event to happen.

A very reliable staff member of the Mental Health Unit didn't arrive for shift one day. The staff tried contacting her, thinking she had mixed up her roster. No one could get in touch with her. After about a week of not arriving for duty, the staff became very concerned as this behaviour was completely out of character. The police were contacted. They reported there had been large withdrawals, from her bank account at several different, automatic teller machines. The police went to her unit and found her body wrapped in plastic. She had suffocated and it was clear she had been murdered. The police found her killer. What a waste of a decent human being.

On another shift I received a call to say two members of nursing staff had been brought to hospital following an apparent drug overdose. The female nurse was dead. I was so shocked. I knew her well from the last hospital I worked at. The male was the nurse who sat on the lounge with the rod wielding man in the Mental Health Unit. He was in a vegetative state from which he never recovered. His family came to collect him and take him home to New Zealand.

The terrible events I was exposed to, I now know are testament to the fact that I was at the doorway into the horrible world of Post-Traumatic Stress Disorder (PTSD). I nearly lost it one night shift when a very senior member of the Emergency Department's nursing staff was brought in dead after drowning in her pool at home. The department was in chaos as the staff decompensated due to the horror of having to care for the body of one of their own. I had to deploy staff left, right and centre to keep the department functioning. Once again, I notified the Executive team member on call (who must by now regard me as a bloody jinx). I instigated the immediate debrief. The Nursing Unit Manager came in to support the staff and allow them to grieve. The Area Health Service counsellor was notified and support networks were established. That consideration didn't appear to apply to the After-Hours Managers though. I drove home after that horrendous shift beyond numb and upset, for I too knew the deceased nurse.

I started having trouble sleeping and devolved into a very dark place. I now recognise I was suffering from a major depressive disorder. Panic attacks and palpitations would overwhelm me. Many times, I would have to leave the inside of my house and escape to the back yard. To me, the inside of the house was a vacuum. My husband would walk outside with me. He has always been so supportive. But living with depression is debilitating for family members too and it has taken its toll on him. I started smoking and drinking again – too much. Alcohol muted my feelings and the world around me. It also allowed me to sleep, albeit badly.

I was becoming fatalistic in my thinking and catastrophising events that while unlikely, to me, seemed very likely. For example, if we had a lot of rain, would the neighbour's house slip off its piers and kill me in my sleep? My dreams were haunted by terror. I would be chased by something or someone, or I would be lost and not able to find my way home, causing me to wake up in a sweat with my heart beating like a jackhammer. Hyperventilating, I would launch out of bed and head out to the back yard, to the fresh air where I could breathe again.

I dreaded going to work for fear of what was going to happen next. It took me all my resolve to get dressed and drive to the hospital. I would be a palpitating wreck by the time I pulled up in the car park. Sometimes it would take me twenty minutes to pluck up the courage to get out of the car. I would wait until the last possible minute to enter the building. At the end of each shift, I couldn't get out of the hospital fast enough.

The relationships between the After-Hours Managers were less than ideal. There was considerable infighting about rosters and work practices. God help you if the bed statement was incorrect; nothing short of a tirade of abuse and criticism would be the response. There was gossiping, back biting and just plain spite. It was all very wearing. It didn't help that there was bugger all support for those of us who worked after hours. We weren't regarded as real managers. It seemed our sole purpose was to keep the ship afloat until the proper managers returned to work.

Every day, I felt like I was going to war. I hated my job. I was disillusioned with nursing and even more so with nurses. I thought I was going mad. It beggars' belief why I stayed in that job. But money and status are enticing demons. I worked shift work in a senior position, so the money was great; it funded a huge mortgage for 3/4 of an acre in a rural village on the outskirts of Sydney at the foot of the beautiful Blue Mountains. We had plenty of money and a great social life. But no amount of money or prestige can outweigh fear and loathing.

I got to a point of absolute hopelessness and was fearful that what I was experiencing today was how my professional life was going to be forever. Jesus! I still had 30 work years until I could retire. God help me, if this was how it was going to be, I needed to get serious about protecting myself. This, I now know, was the time when my tendency towards hypervigilance kicked into gear. Unconsciously, I became watchful for situations that had the potential to lead to adverse outcomes. I would see a situation and immediately go to worst case scenario, which, 99.9% of the time, never came to fruition. I didn't realise I was catastrophising events, perhaps to pre-empt the next horrendous situation that would involve me and cut me off at the knees. Vivid scenarios both real and imagined played in a loop in my brain, over and over again. I couldn't turn them off. They were the thoughts of madness.

I will never forget the day the thought of escape by not living this life anymore occurred to me; If I were dead, the fear and anxiety would go away, what blessed solace that would be.

I would be free again. Calmly and logically, I accepted what I already knew, that my family loved me and that they would grieve for me, but the thought of never having to feel like this ever again was so enticing I began to consider how I could end my life. I can only describe the relief at the prospect of freedom as if I were suddenly showered and encompassed by a golden light. It was so uplifting. I felt like the weight of the world had been removed from my shoulders. Not living this life anymore seemed like one of the best ideas I have ever had.

Sometimes, life gives you a shake to make you stop and reflect and sometimes, it gives you a kick in the arse. I remember the morning I was getting ready for work, when it hit me, Shit! I want to die! I'm going to kill myself. I don't know what shocked me more, the thought of wanting to die or the making of plans to achieve that reality. I needed a plan — now — for I knew what I had to do to make this life I was living go away. In a rare moment of clarity, the reality of my thoughts hit me like a ton of bricks. I ran to the phone and made an appointment with my GP. I remember I just got into the car and drove to the surgery, probably still in my pyjamas and slippers. I was bedraggled, un-showered and a sobbing mess. I will never forget the look of shock on my doctor's face when he saw me. He could tell by the sight of me that I was in a terrible place and while I am while not a fashionista, I am always well-presented and would never leave home without lippie and mascara, except in the event of fire or haemorrhage.

We talked for a long time. I told him I just wanted to be free of this life. I confessed to suicidal ideation and that I had a plan in place to achieve that end. He started me on antidepressants, which like alcohol, muted my feelings and dulled the sharp edges off my life. Seriously, I believe Zoloft should be added to the nation's water supply. I refer to this period in my life as 'the time I fell off my twig.' I started seeing a Clinical Psychologist and slowly life began to fall back into some semblance of order. It was good while it lasted.

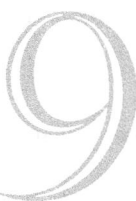

I came to refer to the place where I worked as the 'Hospital from Hell'. The Director of Nursing retired and was succeeded by a woman who was highly intelligent, articulate and an out of the box thinker. She was also very ambitious. Her passion was sailing. She owned a boat and managed the incredible pressures of such a high-powered job as well as sailing the high seas. Thank God! I was saved! I was certain this woman was the answer to improving patient care and making this hospital a better place to work. For a while, that was certainly the case. She was charismatic and beguiling. She was a workaholic and clearly wanted to initiate systems improvement and recruit a team of people who would be her army of achievers. Pick me! Pick me!

She made a huge impression on me as a leader. However, the challenges of this organisation were enough to break anyone. After a couple of years, she moved into the position of Acting Area Director of Nursing. Eventually, the enormity of the struggles of this organisation wore her down. When the time came to convert the Area Director of Nursing job from 'acting' to the appointment of a permanent incumbent, my view was that she was an absolute shoo-in for the job. It's a good think I didn't bet on the outcome.

The Director of Nursing worked impossible hours. When I relieved in the position as Deputy Director of Nursing, I witnessed just how hard she worked during her usual 12-14 hour days. She was an excellent representative for nursing, and it was my view that she deserved to be appointed. However, in troubled organisations, it is impossible not to tread on toes and make enemies.

After all of her contributions not just to the nursing service but to actual patient service delivery, she was notified by a group email transmitted to everyone in the Area Health Service that she had not been successful in her application and that someone else had been appointed. I remember her reaction to this very public, deliberate act of humiliation and her out of character reply, which showcased her embarrassment, disappointment and heartbreak. She responded in turn to the group email with vitriol and fury. I don't know what became of her after that. It is as if she just vanished off the face of the earth. I have searched for her many times through professional channels and social media. Nothing. It is as if she never existed. Another broken nurse. Another casualty of the Hospital from Hell.

From May to June 1999, 3,920 ethnic Albanians arrived in Australia as part of 'Operation Safe Haven'. I had little to no knowledge of these people until they began arriving at the Hospital from Hell. The term 'Kosovo' is an expression that Orthodox Serbians use and the term 'Kosovar' is applied to Muslim Albanians. In 1999, in a war between these two cultures, there were 10,000 killed and 860,000 Kosovo people driven from their homes by the Serbian forces and into neighbouring countries.

The media of course covered the event extensively and compared the scale of the conflict between these two groups of people as not having been seen in Europe since Nazi Germany. The United Nations High Commissioner for Refugees appealed to countries for refugee support. Initially, the (then) Prime Minister of Australia, John Howard, rejected the request of the High Commissioner. However, a high profile, critical media campaign saw an 'about face' and Australia became one of 29 countries to accept the refugees. Of the 840,000 Kosovars who fled their homeland during the conflict, Australia accepted 3,920. This large influx of refugees into Australia was unprecedented. The (then) Minister for Immigration, Philip Ruddock, enacted the 'Temporary Safe Haven' and 'Temporary Protection Refugee Visa Policy' which in a nutshell was a strategic move that restricted the refugees' rights to judicial review, removed human rights protections, and granted the Immigration Minister unprecedented and extraordinary powers to issue or cancel visas. The Australian Safe Haven Visa Policy has been described by Robert Carr of Wollongong University, "As a compassionate intervention with cruel intentions."

I knew nothing about any of this. All I knew was that the Hospital from Hell received a flood of patients with various, sometimes serious health issues or communicable diseases such as tuberculosis. Of course, there were pregnant women who delivered their babies in a strange country with people who didn't speak their language, with midwives and nurses who had no idea of their cultural mores or norms. When I think about it now, I question why as health care professionals we didn't receive education and a thorough briefing about these people and how we could make their transition to Australia less traumatic. Why wasn't there a raft of interpreters available 24 hours per day, seven days a week? Better communication would have made these patients' transition to Australia a little less difficult, and certainly would have made our jobs easier.

Australians for the most part are known as being an easy-going race that live in 'the lucky country' and for most Australians, that is true. Unless, of course, you don't have white skin and aren't a homegrown Aussie. Our treatment of the Kosovars is not so far removed from the appalling treatment by white Australians of Australian First Nations people, who have lived in this country for more than 60,000 years. Captain James Cook arrived here on the 29th April 1770. Those of us of European heritage are the invaders, yet the First Nations population of Australia have horrendous morbidity and mortality statistics, are over-represented in our jails and are treated like second class citizens. It sickens me.

I am ashamed of how policy makers have no real insight into First Nations culture and the importance it plays in their lives. The answer to date has been to keep throwing money at programs to improve First Nations health and wellbeing without any real cultural engagement. Australia is the lucky country — but only if you are white, middle class or above, and pay your taxes.

At the time of Operation Safe Haven, I was 44 years old and while I had experienced racial comments in the past, I had never experienced racial hatred. When the refugees were admitted to the hospital, it became very clear, very quickly, that violence between these people was an everyday part of life which presented a real threat to the other patients and to the staff. To maintain some sort of order in which we could care for these patients without the risk of harm, we spread them to the four corners of the hospital. The strategy was to keep the two groups separate until they were ready to be discharged to Haven Centres where they would complete their stay in Australia.

It was at this time in my life that I finally understood what it would be like to be a First Nations person in this country — disrespected, misunderstood and disadvantaged. I am forever grateful to have been fortunate enough to have been born in Australia — 5th generation — probably from good old English convict stock. I will never accept the hardships imposed upon Australian First Nations people. White Australians removed First Nation children from their families and continue to do so under the guise of Family and Community Services. Their sacred land was stolen from them. They are the true Australians and yet, even today, they continue to be treated like refugees. Australia has a shitty track record for their attitude and lack of generosity towards refugees. I am ashamed every time I see politicians spruiking about policies that will benefit First Nations health and outcomes. How can any race prosper when they are disrespected, culturally dispossessed and dislocated from their sacred land sites? Someone has to care. I do.

In the year 2000 Sydney hosted the Olympic Games. In contrast to Operation Safe Haven this was a time I will always remember with pride. The Olympics was one of the biggest events ever held in Australia with 10,000 athletes and 5,100 officials from 200 countries participating in 28 sporting events. The build up to the 'Games' was electrifying and exciting. Australians may be easy going, but we are also incredibly creative, inventive and know how to put on a good show. At any given time between the 13th of September and the 3rd of October there were an additional 200,000 people in the centre of Sydney between the hours of

12pm and 10pm. Our transport systems, communications and health care preparations won the praise of the world. In fact, the Olympic Health Surveillance System (for athletes, visitors and residents) was lauded as the most comprehensive health preparation system ever established for an Olympic Games.

On the 15th of September the world saw an Opening Ceremony like no other. Sydney put on her best show ever and as a nation we were so proud. The rest of the events went off like clockwork. Even today, the 'Sydney Games' are lauded as the best ever Olympics in modern history.

The Hospital from Hell boasts a large, well equipped Trauma Centre. As After-Hours Managers, our job was to ensure swift triage of any injured athletes or visitors and to protect them from the ever-present media. It was estimated that 15,000 media personnel would cover the Games. If an athlete became injured, they were whisked out of public view, while journalists with hidden cameras sat patiently in the Emergency Department waiting for 'the money shot.' Journalists are creative, I will give them that. Some even had the audacity to pretend to be a weeping relative who needed to be by the bedside of their injured relative. Of course, when the information was conveyed to the patient, they didn't have an Aunty Kobo or Uncle Wilhelm. The 'visitor' would invariably be a devious journalist who would do anything for a story or headline grabbing pictorial evidence. Not on my watch.

The staff and the After-Hours Managers were hypervigilant. A member of our team was set up at triage to ensure any injured athletes, officials or spectators were expedited through the system, and greedy journalists went home empty handed. Managing health care during this time was like being part of a well-oiled machine — and I loved being a part of it.

All too soon, the Olympics were over. I was sad to see the party end. Life took on its everyday face and for me, it was back to working in a large, dysfunctional tertiary hospital. This was an exhausting place to work. Not only because of the sheer size of the place, but because of the unrealistic expectations of the role of the After-Hours Manager, which included rounds of every clinical area to confirm the number of empty beds and to ensure the continued smooth working of the organisation. Any drugs that were out of stock on the ward areas were required to be retrieved from the after-hours pharmacy and be hand delivered to the ward. This could happen many times during a single shift. We walked endless kilometres each and every shift.

I had a standing joke about the pace of work for the After-Hours Managers at this hospital. The yardstick I used to determine the busyness factor was somewhere between chaotic and Oh Jesus! It never got any less hectic than that. At the end of one particular Oh Jesus! busy evening shift, on throbbing feet and very tired legs I left the building, glad as always, to be outside of those walls. In the gloom I saw someone dressed in a nurse's uniform sitting, hunched over, on the steps that led to the car park. I was completely surprised to find it was Monique, the experienced Intensive Care nurse whom I had a lot of time for. She wasn't only an excellent clinician and great patient advocate; she had loads of commonsense and a sense of humour that always made me laugh. I respected her and we had always got on well. When it comes to senior experienced nurses, there are hard arses and then there are really hard arses, Monique fell into the latter category.

I couldn't believe what I was seeing. She was sobbing and distraught. I knew whatever was wrong must have been very bad because she was as tough as they come. I stopped to talk to her. She could hardly speak. Her hand that held a lit cigarette shook like someone with advanced Parkinsonism. I stood quietly beside her until she gained enough composure to be able to speak. This moment is an indelible stamp on my brain. As she explained the scenario, numbness — despite the antidepressants and lessons learned from my Clinical Psychologist — began to take over my body. On the evening shift, Monique had been assigned to care for a woman in her mid-seventies. The patient was postoperatively stable and was discharged ventilated and sedated from the Recovery Room to the Intensive Care Unit. The patient had undergone aorto-bifemoral bypass surgery; a complicated procedure that requires the hands of a skilled vascular surgeon. As part of the patient's care, a Morphine and

Midazolam infusion was commenced via a syringe driver. The volume of the infusion was 50 millilitres. This is a usual part of care for a ventilated patient, to ensure the patient is comfortable and their pain is kept under control. There is a significant risk of over infusing elderly patients with intravenous fluids, which can result in pulmonary oedema (lungs filling up with fluid). To avoid this complication from manifesting itself, a concentrated dose of pain relief is administered in tiny amounts, such as one or two millilitres per hour via a syringe driver over a designated period of time.

At some time during the shift, the on-duty Intensive Care medical staff specialist received a trauma call from the Emergency Department stating an ambulance was enroute with a ventilated young man who had been involved in a motorcycle accident. The patient had sustained serious head injuries and was in a critical condition. The Intensive Care staff specialist alerted the Neurosurgery team. The injured man was rushed to theatre for urgent brain surgery. Unknown to the nursing Team Leader, the Intensive Care doctor had already accepted the patient, who was now in theatre, to come to the Intensive Care Unit postoperatively. If the nursing team leader had been aware she would have pointed out the unit was full to the rafters, there was nowhere to put the patient, nor was there a member of nursing staff available to care for him. The Intensive Care doctor was aware of this fact when he accepted the patient. It was a simple matter of mathematics, to accept this patient into the Intensive Care Unit, the bed occupancy needed to be reduced by one existing patient in order to free up a bedspace and a nurse.

Monique could barely speak. I remember joining her on the step, and after some time, she advised me she had witnessed the Intensive Care staff specialist go to her patient's bedside and pull the curtains closed. Within a couple of minutes, alarms started blaring from the bedspace. The doctor walked out from behind the curtain dusting his hands together. The staff all responded to resuscitate the patient. He told Monique and the rest of the staff, "No resus," and walked away.

Like a robot stuck in a loop, Monique told me she just kept saying, "What the fuck just happened? What the fuck just happened?"

The patient had undergone very complicated vascular surgery. Monique was hysterical by this stage.

"She was ventilated and yes she was in her 70's, but she was stable, she wasn't dying!"

It was as if Monique was alone, talking to herself. "She was stable. We had just started the Morph' and Midaz' syringe driver. She was comfortable and stable."

I remember she paused, and like a marathon runner she was breathless. "Kath, when I went to the bedside, the syringe driver was empty. That bastard had taken the syringe from the driver and pushed the whole thing. It was empty. That is why she had a brady (bradycardic) arrest. He killed her."

There had been sufficient medication in the syringe to deliver micro doses of pain relief for the next 24 hours. With no resuscitation permitted, the patient died because Morphine depresses the respiratory centre in the brain. A lethal dose like the one this patient received was responsible for her death. Not long after that, the staff specialist was informed by the Neurosurgeon that the young man in theatre had head injuries that were too severe to survive the surgery. He had died on the table.

Monique was inconsolable. It was surreal. It was like being in a terrible heartbreaking movie. The only difference was, this was real. This had really happened. She kept saying over and over that the patient was not dying, that she was stable and that she would have recovered. The patient's life had been deliberately terminated based on resource allocation. Monique told me this particular medical officer frequently voiced objection to the allocation of prohibitively expensive, limited, Intensive Care resources on the aged. As she sobbed, Monique confessed there were other nurses in the Intensive Care Unit who held suspicions about this doctor and his unethical, ageist attitude. This was not the first time elderly patients had died unexpectedly when he was on duty. Panicked she told me after her patient had died and had been removed to the mortuary, the Intensive Care Staff Specialist had started hanging around a bedspace occupied by another aged patient. Monique predicted the patient would also be dead by morning.

I was shocked to my very core. At no stage did I not believe what Monique was telling me. I rang my counterpart on night shift and relayed the information as it had been given to me. I also informed her of Monique's predication about the other patient. I hung up and rang the Intensive Care Team Leader on shift and advised him of the potential threat to the patient. I also advised him if the patient was dead in the morning, I would go to the police. Sounds fantastic and unbelievable? Absolutely, and yet it happened.

I finally arrived late and in truth, I didn't recall the drive home. I told my husband what had transpired. It was at that moment when fear unlike anything I have ever experienced, overwhelmed me. I couldn't breathe. I know now, that was the moment I ceased to function as a rational human being. The fear owned me.

The next day, after no sleep, I went to work on the afternoon shift. The first thing I did was to enquire about the other aged patient Monique had held concerns for. Thankfully, the night duty After-Hours Manager had assigned a nurse to be at the patient's bedside at all times – no exceptions — and if the staff held any concerns about the Intensive Care staff specialist interfering with the patient's treatment, she was to be notified immediately. The patient survived the shift and was stepped down to a ward bed the next morning. She will never know just how close she came to prematurely meeting her maker.

I rang the Director of Nursing and requested a meeting with her. After I informed her of Monique's confession, she looked up at me and said, "You need to be very careful about what you say."

She nodded her head towards the door. "This meeting is over."

I was bewildered as I had been careful to recount the story as it had been told to me. It was clear she already knew what had happened. She kicked me out of her office.

When a patient dies within 24 hours of surgery, a coronial inquiry is required. All tubes and lines must be left in place and an autopsy is performed to determine the cause of death. This is one of the many concerns I still harbour to this day about this event. Firstly, Morphine and Midazolam are restricted Schedule 8 and Schedule 4 drugs. They are accountable substances which by law are required to be signed out of the dangerous drug cupboard in the presence of two staff members, one of whom must be a registered nurse. Residual amounts of these drugs that are not required by the patient are likewise required to be destroyed and documented as accounted for, in the presence of two staff members. The syringe driver attached to Monique's patient was empty within a short time after commencement of the infusion. To this day, I question why this anomaly was not a glaring red flag? Both Monique and I talked with the Director of the Intensive Care Unit. She dismissed Monique's claim out of hand and treated us like we had concocted this fantastic story for reasons known only to us.

My stress levels working at this hospital were off the Richter scale. One Friday evening shift, I experienced my second episode of SVT. My heart rate was around 200 beats per minute. I was breathless, panting and dizzy. I rang the Director of Nursing to advise what was happening and that I needed to see her. She advised me to come and see her on Monday! I was the only After-Hours Manager on duty so it wasn't as though I could just pack up and leave, although every synapse in my brain screamed for me to do so. The Director of Nursing should have suggested she call one of the other After-Hours Managers in and relieve me of duty. I spent the rest of the shift hiding in the office with the door locked. I did my job by radar via the phone and by delegation. Professional responsibility over self-preservation. Just plain dumb.

It was around this time that a Director of one of the hospital Divisions stepped up into the role of hospital Director of Nursing. By now, I was well and truly coming unravelled at the seams. I was hypervigilant and paranoid, conjuring in my mind scenarios of adverse outcomes for patients. Sleep deprivation was a really big part of my devolution into the darkest of dark places. I was a slave to terror that would ultimately jettison me into abject decompensation. I hated going to work. Not only that, all the joy was sucked out of my life. I was so depressed that I didn't even consider doing the most obvious, logical thing – to resign and get the hell out of there. The madness of depression became my life. I had a mortgage to pay and a family to feed. It was not an option for me to be without a job, I had to keep the wolf from the door. Just keep going. Just keep going. Just keep going.

10

Monique was damaged by the death of her patient; beyond broken. In fact, she became obsessed, cornering staff at every opportunity, in an effort to convince them that what she had alleged was true. Like me, she became preoccupied by the events of that night. As is human nature, if there is a possibility that by association someone will become embroiled in an adverse outcome, they will simply stop listening and walk away. Monique was ostracised by her colleagues but she just couldn't let it go. What had happened to her patient went against everything she believed in as a professional nurse and as a decent human being.

It soon became apparent that she was getting too close to hitting a nerve. The Acting Director of Nursing alleged Monique was a drug affected nurse, the purpose of which was to provide a smoke screen to explain her obsessive behaviour and to detract from further inquiry into the patient's death. This accusation was made without any evidence of drug abuse or drug theft. The Acting Director of Nursing lodged a formal complaint against

Monique to the (then) professional regulatory body for nurses —The Nurses and Midwives Board of NSW. This action achieved the desired intention — to shut Monique up. Shame and disgrace hung from her like a mantle. She was professionally humiliated and her faith in human goodness was in tatters. The endgame was achieved; she was no longer able to function. She went on extended leave, in disgrace, and didn't come back. Problem solved.

The events of working at the Hospital from Hell, the loss of Monique to an uncertain future and violation of so many of the tenets of a professional nurse became overwhelming. I realised I too was broken by the events of the past, like a marionette with severed strings. I wasn't just broken I was permanently broken. The scales in my professional life had tipped too far. After a sleepless night, I couldn't stop crying; I was back in that dark place where the beckon of death...suicide, was enticing. All I wanted was to follow those thoughts, like a child to Pan's flute.

This episode of suicidal ideation was not as stark as it had been the first time when I devolved into the darkness. My life was permanently muted by the effects of antidepressants. But even through the fog, I realised I was in real trouble. Yes, suicide is an escape, but my family, how would they ever come to terms with the fact that I took my own life? I am the glue that keeps the family together. The pain I would cause my family would be much greater than anything I had ever experienced. For a blink in time, reason reared its head. My warrior spirit arose like a phoenix from the ashes and I went to see my GP again. We talked for a long time. He insisted I not return to work as clearly the impact of my job had severely affected my mental health. He increased the dose of anti-depressants, informed my Clinical Psychologist of the events leading up to my relapse then completed the paperwork for Workers Compensation, citing my mental health status as attributable to workplace-induced acute psychological distress.

I was unable to bring myself to drive to the hospital to submit the forms. I felt like a coward, but I had nothing in reserve to give me the strength to drive there and meet with the Acting Director of Nursing face-to-face. I faxed the documents and tried not to care that she would think I was a weak and spineless human being. Fear consumed me. Anxiety, palpitations and insomnia became my constant companions. Weeks later, after the paperwork was submitted, I was notified in an official capacity by the Area Health Service that nurses do not suffer from psychological distress. It was stated that the distress I was experiencing was a manifestation of a pre-existing mental illness. In other words, I was mad.

I stayed at home, vacillating between feeling like I was getting a grip on my life to being paralysed by fear and loathing by the thought that this state may well be how the rest of my life was going to be. In truth, I exhausted my husband with his constant worry about me, a condition that has remained with him to this day. I regret that I am responsible for that. He is a wonderful, caring, loving man. No one should have to be afraid to go to work and return home to find their spouse dead by their own hand. Every day, while I was at home and the children were at school, he would ring me at least twenty times a day. If I happened to miss one of his calls, he would become frantic and keep ringing until I answered. He was chronically tired, slept poorly and my situation consumed his life. I am responsible for the fear and depression he experiences today. For that I am deeply regretful.

Prior to all of these events, we had a great group of friends and an enviable social life. We loved being part of a rural village, living on lots of land with a lovely house, hens, dogs, cats, fish, plenty of money and happiness. Depression is a dark nebulous thing that extends its tendrils trying to draw others under its shadowy wings. When I became depressed and acopic; the sound of our friends' retreating feet was deafening. Now, we were alone.

This was an extremely difficult time. There was just my husband, myself and our two young children. Neither of our families lived close by. It was just us because I had exhausted all of our friends. Our isolation was a result of my fixation on the events at the Hospital from Hell. This was a wake-up call for me. I was desperate to find a means to find me again. Because the person I was at this point in my life was nothing like the person I knew myself to be.

This was when I realised the value of meditation. For a very long time I struggled to control my over-thinking, frantic brain, long enough to try to find a place where I could find peace and reason through what was and wasn't real. I attended regular Clinical Psychologist appointments to try and put the pieces of my life back together. Many times, I resented that person sitting opposite me with the obligatory sympathetic expression and soft-spoken voice. How do textbook verbatim answers help me to cope with the life sucking fears that had consumed my existence? I guess by attending these appointments, somewhere in my brain I ticked a box that affirmed I was not a failure and that I was making positive steps towards making a better future for me; a future where that relentless voice in my brain that reinforces negative thoughts of hopelessness, would be silenced.

After weeks of struggle, it came to me. I have always been an eternally poetic soul, who finds joy in words. Ironically, it was a litany from the Bene Gesserit witches — Dune (the movie) that put things into perspective for me.

"I must not fear.

Fear is the mind-killer.

Fear is the little-death that brings total obliteration.

I will face my fear.

I will permit it to pass over me and through me.

And when it has gone past, I will turn the inner eye to see its path.

Where the fear has gone there will be nothing.

Only I will remain."

During one of my daily meditation sessions that were slowly becoming less frantic and more surreal, the words 'fear is the mind-killer', played over and over in my brain, when clarity revealed reality and lit the path for my journey back to sanity. I use this mantra every day. In fact, it is written on a board in my kitchen. People often ask me about it. I always say, if you let what you are afraid of stop you from living your life, then the fear will have won.

I was finding myself again, however my paid leave was running out. Before I knew it, my leave balances were exhausted and the wolf was back clawing at the door. I had two choices; either go back to work or lose the house. The fear of failing my family was as great as my fear of going back to the front line and facing life at that bloody horrible hospital again.

I contacted the now formally appointed Director of Nursing and set a date and time to meet with her. I recall on the day of the meeting; I vomited in the car park from hyperventilation and anxiety. I just kept putting one foot in front of the other, until after what seemed like the longest time, I was outside her office. I felt like I was in a vacuum. I couldn't breathe, there was no air in the room and I was a lather of sweat. I went to the bathroom, wet some paper hand towels, sat on the lid of a toilet and placed the wad of wet paper on the back of my neck, closed my eyes and reached into my mind.

"I must not fear.

Fear is the mind-killer.

Fear is the little-death that brings total obliteration.

I will face my fear.

I will permit it to pass over me and through me.

And when it has gone past, I will turn the inner eye to see its path.

Where the fear has gone there will be nothing.

Only I will remain."

I left the bathroom and returned to sit on a chair outside of her office. Calm and peace had found me. The door opened and the Director of Nursing's face was a mask of kindness and sympathy which rapidly changed when I spoke about suicidal ideation and the challenges I faced coming to work again. Clearly, she saw me as someone who had the potential to end my life, leaving a damning paper trail. I clearly represented a situation that could very easily implode her newly promoted, stellar career. Thinking on her feet, she asked me if I would be interested in utilising my significant knowledge of policy and procedure writing to assist her with a back log of work. She requested I meet her at 8am the following Monday, which would give her sufficient time to construct the brief of what the position would entail.

I drove home feeling like a miracle had happened. I didn't have to go back to work as an After-Hours Manager! I was out of the firing line! Everything at last was going to work out and life would be good again, the way it used to be. There was a time when I used to have an unfailing belief in the goodness of humanity — today, not so much. I wanted so much to believe the worst was behind me and that the Director of Nursing would support me.

How skilful she was. Like the bansuri player who mesmerises a snake, she enticed me into the rhythm of her dance.

I remember the weekend before I was scheduled to meet with the Director of Nursing, I was busy clacking away at the keyboard, making notes and references, swotting up on contemporary health policy and procedure templates and future directions. I wanted to be prepared to create worthwhile documents, to be energised and ready to offer my contribution to the organisation and celebrate my return to the workplace. On the following of Monday, after doing an hour of meditation while sitting in the car park, I presented to the Director of Nursing's office. She took me to an abandoned building where there was a desk, a telephone and various stacks of paperwork. It became clear to me over the next few weeks that the tasks set for me were inconsequential with no timeline for completion.

The reality of my situation became clear to me. I had been deliberately isolated and marginalised under the guise of a supported framework in which I could return to work. Within a short time, all of the correspondence was sorted. The only tasks for me to complete were the crossword puzzles in the newspapers I took to work. I slowly relinquished the dream of finally being able to find my way back into the 'real' nursing managerial workforce. I felt such a fool to have fallen for the Director of Nursing's false concern for me. The true sucker punch came when it finally dawned on me that she never had any intention of allowing me to take up any position again.

It was clear to me that I was regarded as a liability. The Director of Nursing had done what the Area Health Service had advised her to do and turned the tables on me. To the profession, it would appear that she had gone out of her way to create a position for me whereby I was out of the firing line and given the opportunity to recover. Any complaints from me regarding isolation or marginalisation would be interpreted as ingratitude. The tendrils of darkness that I had thought had been blown away, reached out and completely consumed me again. Give the lady a medal.

I needed to get the hell out of this hospital, I knew that, but one of the tenets of my middle-class upbringing was that one didn't give up a job unless there was another one to go to. It was deemed irresponsible to do otherwise. I guess my question is, does that rule still apply if the job is causing harm? As in other areas of my life, 'roots' are very important to me. I was more than ready to put down employment roots - to see out the years I have left until I am due to retire. At this time, was nearly 50 years of age, but roots were not going to happen at the Hospital from Hell.

I am a bloody good nurse. How could this situation have been allowed to occur? God help me, once again my sense of social justice burned in my soul. Are the words in the NSW Health Code of Conduct just lip service? Health care professionals have a duty of care to their patients; as does NSW Health to its staff.

The warrior in me once again sprang to life. If I was going to go out, I would go out fighting. I wrote to the Director of Nursing and advised it was my intention to seek legal counsel on the grounds the Area Health Service had failed to provide a safe workplace and had failed me in its duty of care. That put the cat amongst the pigeons.

I am articulate and always do my homework before engaging in any battle. After long and tedious communications back and forth with the Area Health Service, I made it abundantly clear that I knew my rights and was not going to be brow beaten or chased away. Again, I was informed there had never been a successful lawsuit by a nurse for psychological distress. Apparently that situation only arises if the person is a police officer or a soldier, which is ironic because every day at this hospital felt like going to war.

I still went to work every day to the abandoned building, just to keep the mortgage paid. I was like a robot. Each morning, I would go onto auto pilot and do nothing, because that was all I had to do. I was emotionally, physically and professionally exhausted.

The lack of worthwhile work and workplace involvement was a constant reminder to me of my lack of value to the organisation and to the profession. This was a time of torture for me; a violation of everything about the profession of nursing that I believed in. Out of the blue, without any prior conversation, came an official letter bearing the Area Health Service's logo. I was offered a paltry few thousand dollars, in essence, to get rid of me. There was a legal proviso that I sign a waiver that would prevent me from ever bringing legal action against the Hospital from Hell or the Area Health Service in the future.

I wasn't thinking straight. All I could see was a means of escape from this place of nightmares and money to offer me some breathing space to find another job. To my very great detriment, I signed the documents then tendered my resignation.

On my last day, I returned to the After-Hours Managers office and copied all of the emails between myself and the Director of Nursing. Someone must have seen me and given the manager the heads up. As I walked away from the office, she met me in the corridor and asked me what I was doing. I advised I was taking my correspondence with me. She blocked my way and advised I was not permitted to remove Area Health Service property from the premises. I side stepped her and kept walking, fully expecting to be intercepted by Security at any moment. I just put my head down and put one foot in front of the other. When I got to the car park, I was so tremulous I couldn't put the key in the ignition. All I could imagine was big burly security officers descending upon me like Storm Troopers. I finally managed to get the car going. My mouth was filled with vomit. I thought I might pass out. Jesus! I was unemployed, but I was free.

The blood money from the Area Health Service dwindled rapidly, but the mortgage got paid. All too soon, the dollars and time were running out and I needed a job—now! In my career, I had never had a problem securing employment. However, time was of the essence, so I joined a nursing agency while I applied for full time jobs. I knew a number of staff from this agency when I worked as an After-Hours Manager while at the Hospital from Hell. I had always found this agency to be reliable and efficient.

It was 2002. In that year I lodged 64 job applications. How naive was I? Some of the applications apparently didn't even warrant an acknowledgement. The rest all started with "Dear... Thank you for your application. I regret to inform you that you have been unsuccessful..."

What the hell was going on? I applied for jobs that I was eminently qualified for and with the experience to perform to a very high standard, yet I didn't get invited to interview. I also applied for jobs that were below my expected pay grade, just to get a permanent job. I still didn't get any invitations to interview.

Finally, a letter arrived confirming an interview date for an After-Hours Manager's position at a peripheral hospital. Thank God. At last, I could leave agency nursing and find stability in a permanent job. I had worked a night shift before the scheduled interview but had done my homework on the demographics of the hospital and the wider service it belonged to. I arrived 20 minutes early, as is my practice, to go over my notes. My paperwork was in order, I was confident and well prepared. The interview began ordinarily enough with the usual questions about my understanding of the role, the obligatory conflict resolution question and what qualities did I bring to the role that would benefit the hospital? It was then that the convenor of the panel looked at me through slitted eyes and said, "I know who you are and what you did. You spoke out and caused a whole lot of trouble. I would never employ you here at this hospital or anywhere else. Don't bother to ever apply to this hospital again. There will never be a job for you here."

Profound silence. I didn't know what to do. I just sat there, stunned. My tired brain tried to convince me that what I had just heard was a sleep deprived aberration and that I had misunderstood. The converor gathered the pieces of paper in front of him, tapped them into a tidy heap and left the room. Jesus! I had been invited to interview so he could have his pound of flesh and tell me exactly what he thought of me. There was never any real consideration of my application, the interview was simply an opportunity for him to vent his spleen.

    The faces of the panel members confirmed they had been pre-informed of the end game of this interview. At least they had the good grace to look uncomfortable and embarrassed. I stood, shook their hands, thanked them for their time and went out to the car park. I got into my car and sobbed. That was when this girl from the country realised her career would never be the same again.

11

I soon learned it takes balls to work as an agency nurse/midwife. It had been 16 years since I had last worked as a clinician. To be a nurse/midwife in New South Wales, the current authority to practice was issued by the (then) Nurses Registration Board. The same applied to agency nurses/midwives. From that point onward, achieving bookings for shifts was a lottery.

An agency nurse is a gap filler; a nurse who will bring the staffing allocation for the shift up to the required numbers. There is no guarantee of level of experience or competence nor was there a guarantee of the 'like for like' principle. If a registered nurse calls in sick and there is a less expensive option, for example an endorsed enrolled nurse or an assistant in nursing, that option will often be taken up. The numbers will be restored but very often, the skill mix is skewed, which can impact directly upon patient safety and patient outcomes.

For me, there was very little job satisfaction attached to working as an agency nurse/midwife. The work was all about going where there was a staffing deficit, which equates to rarely caring for the same patients two shifts in a row. The harsh reality was the work was about getting booked for shifts and to put money in the bank. Getting booked for shifts was high risk and very much hit and miss. It was paramount that the nurse/midwife proves they were competent, reliable and not going to create any grief for the employing hospital or particularly for the after-hours managers. Agency nurses compete against the employing hospital's cheque book. If an agency nurse/midwife was unreliable, or a problem, there would be no shifts forthcoming. Play the game or not, at your very great peril.

To get through every day as an agency nurse/midwife, I had to pretend life was a box of birds. This was a time in my life when I grasped with great certainty how very depressed people throw themselves off cliffs; leaving family and co-workers behind, bewildered as to the reasons why. Depressed people assume glamour, that is, they put on a happy face for the benefit of those around them. Depression is an insidious condition that has many facades. I believe to survive, depressed people must appear as described by J. M. Barrie in the children's book Peter Pan, to have found their 'happy thoughts.' I had no choice. I had to work. I had to portray myself as happy, confident and amenable. I am a highly competent nurse, so no problem there. But no one could know how I really was in terms of the panic, anxiety and bone crushing depression I suffered. If the owners of the agency got wind of just how damaged I was after the events and consequences of being an After-Hours Manager at the Hospital from Hell, I would have remained on their staffing register, but I would never have been booked for any shifts. I needed to keep my head down and my mouth shut.

After I joined the agency, I was fortunate enough to be placed in maternity wards. This was logical, given my extensive history as a midwife, but more importantly, this experience gave me the chance to ease back into the clinical environment.

My first few shifts were on the postnatal ward. I had forgotten how lovely it was to spend time teaching new mothers about breast feeding and baby care. However, the face of midwifery had changed a great deal in the time I had been off working in non-midwifery jobs. This was fast paced work with too few beds, too few midwives and too many patients. Nurses and midwives are resourceful; they have to be, to manage the volume of the work. They are also highly critical of colleagues who don't get their work finished by the end of their shift. Cutting corners is a fact of life — as long as the outcome equals the actual way the procedure is supposed to be done — so no win, no foul. But some cut corners put patients at high risk of an adverse outcome.

I recall working in a private hospital where one particular midwife who was usually in-charge of the shift advised me she was going on her 'break'. I asked what needed to be done for her patients while she was off the ward. She waved her hand at me and said, "All good, nothing to do. I will fix everything when I get back from my break."

She returned to the ward from her break (sleep) three hours later. Just before dawn, one of her patients buzzed. I knew this particular midwife was in a room with a woman who was having difficulty breast feeding so I answered the buzzer. The patient, who had recently undergone a caesarean section, requested pain relief. I checked her chart to see what I could administer, when I noticed the hourly observations that were due while the midwife was on her break were all complete. Welcome to radar observations.

The ideal nurse that agencies seek is a clinician who has a broad range of experience, a jack of all trades so to speak; a nurse who can slot into any clinical environment and get the job done. The greater the range of experience, the more shifts. I realised if I was going to get enough work to keep my household afloat, I needed to spread my wings and accept shifts outside of maternity. There are lean times for agency work (the long Christmas period, public holidays and operating theatre down times) when there are not enough shifts to go round. I needed to increase my potential to get shifts. I discussed my proposal with the agency and my areas of work preference expanded exponentially. Initially, I accepted shifts on medical wards and surgical wards which were well within my scope of practice; as was Paediatrics, which I begrudgingly took despite the still vivid memory of that poor burned child. However, this ward didn't have patients with that level of acuity so I ended up enjoying the shifts I worked there.

I don't know, maybe I got cocky, or maybe I just inadvertently slid into that erroneous mentality that if you are a registered nurse, then you are competent to engage in the care of patients of any degree of acuity. I found myself caught between a rock and a hard place. I was offered a night shift in an Intensive Care Unit at a Sydney hospital. I am not an Intensive Care nurse. I have never portrayed myself as having those skills. But to say no to a shift usually was followed by a 'quiet period' in terms of future shifts. I am not saying this was a retaliatory tactic used by the agency to punish nurses who refuse shifts, but it seemed like it to me at the time. The last thing I needed was to get off-side with the agency, plus I needed the money. With trepidation, I accepted the shift.

I remember being anxious and just hoped to God that I would not bring anyone to harm and that the 10-hour shift went quickly. Should I have refused the shift, knowing I was going to be working in Intensive Care? Possibly. It is funny how one can rationalise things to validate decision making.

When I accepted the shift, I knew, as an agency nurse, I would be considered the most junior nurse on shift and would be allocated the least complicated patient. Of course, there would be experienced nurses on shift I could go to if I had questions or if I required clarification. To my great relief, I was allocated a patient whose care was well within my scope of practice. But ironically, it wasn't my patient or his care that was the issue for me on this shift.

There was an elderly man lying in a bed at the side of the unit. Grieving relatives sat behind privacy curtains surrounding his bed. The previous shift at handover advised the patient had presented to hospital with a lung tumour and had been to surgery. He had subsequently developed an abscess in his chest and was now very unwell and too unstable to return to theatre to drain the abscess.

That is when I saw it. On the X-ray viewer light box there was a chest film with this patient's details on it. The patient did have a massive collection in his chest. He also had a piece of surgical gauze in there. The Raytec thread that is in all operating theatre consumables was highly visible to anyone who knew what they were looking at. The advocate in me urged me to tell these people the truth about why their relative had developed the abscess in his chest and that was the reason he was deteriorating. But how could I tell them? The man was going to die regardless and the relatives were already grieving. To inform them of what I knew would only exacerbate their distress. Yes, they could have gotten legal counsel and yes, they probably would have won a settlement, but it would have cost them a great deal to see justice done and the grey-haired man who lay in the bed would still be dead. The only winners in this situation would be the lawyers.

I returned to my patient's bedside and made him as comfortable as possible. By the end of the shift, the old man had passed. His relatives were with him, sobbing their last goodbyes. I grabbed my bag, kept my head down and avoided looking at the X-ray viewer again.

This shift taught me that advocacy has many faces. It is never easy to speak up, because, the ripple effect can be devastating, which would certainly have been the case for this family. In this instance, I advocated for them by maintaining my silence and not exacerbating their grief. I am comfortable that I didn't tell them, for where was the gain? The patient was dead and nothing was going to change that.

I now recognise that by working outside of maternity I was lulled into a false sense of security. I recall the time the agency contacted me about a shift in the same hospital where I had worked many maternity shifts, but this shift was again in Intensive Care. What a quandary. If I refused the shift, the potential for not being considered for future shifts was a reality. I kept thinking about the previous Intensive Care shift and acquiesced to the prospect of continued shift offers and the pressure of the dollar. I accepted the shift.

The agency assured me I would be allocated a patient(s) within my scope of practice and that I would be well supported by the experienced Intensive Care Nurses. Again, I was just plain naive.

I was assigned to a patient who had a multi-resistant Staphylococcal aureus infection (Golden Staph) which meant I had to be gowned, gloved and masked the entire time I was in his isolation room. He was extremely unwell with fever, and he had a tracheotomy which required suctioning every hour. This involved sliding a small plastic tube attached to a suction machine down the man's breathing tube to draw the secretions from his lungs. I had never cared for a person with a tracheotomy in my entire career. The sum total of my knowledge of tracheotomies was from what I had read in textbooks during my general training, close to 30 years ago. I immediately informed the nursing Team Leader on shift of my complete lack of experience in caring for these types of patients. My honesty was rewarded with an eye roll as she regarded me as if I were an imbecile. I will never forget her words. "Just get on with it. We're full to the rafters and every other patient here is sicker than him. There is no one else I can swap you with." Then she sneered at me, "And don't even think about going home. It's a trachy for God's sake! It doesn't get much easier than that!" She flounced off, shaking her head.

This was a time before mobile phones were commonplace, and before the internet became part of our everyday lives. I spoke to other staff members to bring myself up to speed on how to appropriately care for this patient and prayed he would still be alive in the morning. I attended his observations and suctioning religiously, every hour, on the hour.

Just before dawn, the patient became feverish. I informed the Team Leader who spoke with the Intensive Care Specialist on duty. The Team Leader came into the room and suctioned the tracheotomy tube. A large amount of secretions were extracted. She accused me of not suctioning the patient. At this point, the patient informed her that I had suctioned his tracheotomy tube every hour. The Team Leader finished the suctioning stormed out of the room, saying, "Oh well, then I guess this is just a case of incompetence."

Handover to the morning shift was at 7am. I grabbed my bag and left the Intensive Care Unit. I cried all the way home and the guilt I felt about not suctioning the patient's tracheotomy tube more vigorously was crushing and long lasting. No number of shifts or dollars was worth risking a patient's life or my mental health.

In the year 2000 there were just over 224,500 enrolled nurses and registered nurses and midwives in Australia; but it is a small world. Word had gotten out about my involvement with Monique's ICU patient.

Out of the blue, I was contacted by Narissa, who was an After-Hours Manager I had previously worked with and held her own grave concerns about patient safety. She was also consumed by these concerns. Unbeknown to me, she had also contacted Meadhbh and Yanaha, the theatre Clinical Nurse Specialists to discuss their concerns regarding patient care and patient outcomes.

Anyone who knows nurses and midwives, knows we can 'talk shop' until the cows come home. Narissa arranged for us all to meet, where we willingly shared our concerns about poor patient outcomes, unexpected patient deaths and our suspicions. The one time I met with Narissa, Meadhbh and Yanaha, it didn't occur to me that Narissa had brought us together because she had her own agenda. At the meeting, she was animated, highly agitated and obsessive about the adverse events she had experienced. Her fury was palpable as she relayed the attempts she had made to speak to the management of the facility where she worked.

Narissa's recounted experiences of reporting adverse events mirrored mine — no one was listening. I do believe she was a staunch patient advocate and that she did everything in her power to try and get answers and to protect patients from harm. The toll of those events and her exposure to our collective experiences affected her badly. She became somewhat paranoid and unreservedly distrusting of the healthcare system. We discussed at length my experience with Monique and the patient in Intensive Care and the later consequences for me as a direct result of doing the job I was paid to do, while trying to pursue the truth.

Not long after the meeting where we had all very candidly discussed our extreme concerns about adverse patient outcomes, I was driving home from an agency night shift at a hospital on the outskirts of Sydney. I was aware that Narissa had already been on air several times, sharing conversations about her healthcare concerns with AM radio talk back legend, Alan Jones. I took a keen interest in her conversations with him on his morning program. He is well known, opinionated, controversial and very right wing. It was good that I solely worked night shifts as I never missed a segment. I have to say, I admired Narissa's strength and commitment. She took a no-holds-barred approach. She was passionate in her delivery, and it was clear she advocated for what she believed in. Then it happened.

Live on air, Narissa started discussing my experience with the patient in Intensive Care, but her recount of what actually happened was exaggerated and factually incorrect. I was stunned. Now, put it down to sleep deprivation or exhaustion from the years of nursing's knives being plunged into my back but something just snapped. I parked the car on a misty football oval and pulled out my mobile phone. My fingers sped across the keypad as I dialled the radio station. I spoke to the operator and told her who I was and the reason for my call. She suddenly became very excited. Breathlessly, she asked if I minded if she put me on hold. I didn't care; I was numb.

My heart was hammering in my chest when there was a sudden interruption to the background music and a much younger woman spoke. She said she was the program manager or some such thing. I will give her this, she was one of those people who, when she chatted, made you feel like you are the only person in the world she cared about. She finally got around to asking me to repeat what I had told the operator. I told her who I was, what position I held at the time of the death of the patient Monique had reported to me, and what I knew to be the truth. My recount of the events deviated significantly from that which Narissa, minutes before, had declared as fact. The program manager if I was prepared to speak on air about it to Alan Jones.

I was like a stunned mullet. My brain was parked in neutral and not one neural synapse enacted any sort of warning. I didn't even think about it, I just said yes. Within 10 minutes, I was on air with Alan Jones. What I didn't know then, was that Narissa had a huge following on this program. It was never my intention to embarrass her by contradicting her statement, nor did I realise that by correcting her declarations, I was unwittingly exacerbating public concern for the state of Health in New South Wales. It was important to me that the truth be heard. I felt I owed it to the patient and her relatives.

I relayed the information as it was given to me by Monique — which was no hardship, as those words were then and will be forever more be burned into my brain. To say Alan Jones was incredulous would be an understatement. To say that he believed every word I had said was absolute. I finished the conversation, and the program manager came back on the line, enacting her charming ways as she thanked me for my participation in the program. She asked for my contact details, which thanks to my sleep deprived, stunned brain, I recounted as requested. How naive was I?

I had just spoken out not just on radio but on national radio to the number one AM radio program in Australia! In truth, I was a little excited because maybe someone would care enough to investigate Monique's claims which at no time I had ever doubted. I was relieved that finally the truth would be uncovered. My excitement and sense of relief was short lived.

All hell broke loose. NSW Health went into meltdown. I had not long arrived home, bleary eyed and tired, when John Laws, perhaps Australia's most famous radio announcer, phoned me on my landline. He was the undisputed king of talk back radio in Australia. He was known as 'The Golden Tonsils' and had a reputation for being brutal to his callers. I remember as he spoke to me, he sounded alarmed, but there was also a note of scepticism to his tone. He asked me why I didn't just go to the management of the hospital and declare what had been reported to me by

Monique and leave the matter to be handled as per protocol. I advised I did go to management—more than once. I advised him I had acted as per protocol as an After-Hours Manager and that the game didn't play out after that.

The crashing reality of what I had done, by speaking to the media, hit me like a ton of bricks. He asked me, "Well what happens now?"

I replied, "As a nurse manager, my career is over."

His voice changed after that. In my heart I know he believed what I had said was true. He also knew that I was correct in my assumptions. My career as a manager was over. Little did I know.

The next thing I knew, national radio was on my doorstep and Australia heard my truth. I was inundated with calls from various media outlets, in particular, a young journalist from a Sydney newspaper. We met and discussed my experiences. I gave him Monique's name but I had no contact details for her. The journalist contacted the hospital regarding the information I had given him. He was informed the requested medical records of the patient could not be found. Of course, when this finding became public, the records were miraculously accounted for.

As is the way of the media, no opportunity for sensationalism is ever missed. I was asked to go on-air again to speak to the deceased patient's relatives. The media have no shame — whatever it takes to sell papers is the price paid. The relatives of the deceased woman in Intensive Care had been informed by the hospital that the patient died as a result of postoperative complications. This was technically true; she had died as a result of a bradycardic arrest; I guess they forgot to mention that the patient's heart stopped because she was murdered. The family members harboured great guilt and anguish because they had not been physically at their mother's bedside. They had contacted the hospital many times for progress reports on their mother's post operative progress. Each time they were reassured the surgery had gone well, and that she was stable. They didn't live close to Sydney and had there been any concerns at all, they would have immediately made arrangements to be by her bedside. It is a shame they didn't, the patient perhaps would have survived.

I told the relatives everything I knew on national radio (I guess I was good for ratings that day). They thanked me for my courage and for the truth. When I got off the phone, there was a dead space in my chest, like there had been an apocalypse and I was the sole survivor on the planet. The emptiness and overwhelming sense of loneliness was crushing. I felt no sense of relief that the dead woman's relatives finally knew the truth. Did it do any of us any good? No. They would forever more feel guilty about not being at their mother's bedside, while I, felt like Judas, because the real truth was so much less palatable than to have lost their mother through postoperative complications.

The only winner that day was the media. As participants in that phone call, we were nothing more than ratings fodder. I know now, that that was the day the collective heels of the profession of nursing clicked together as they turned their backs and shunned me. I was no longer entitled to be included in the esprit de corps. I had committed a cardinal sin; I had spoken out and made public an extreme adverse outcome.

Life became a blur. I was overwhelmed by life and twice I suspended my candidature for the Master of Health Management [hons]. This degree was comprised of two course-work units and then a thesis by research. I stood no chance of producing any work that was remotely close to an acceptable academic standard.

The salary of an agency nurse (then) was about $50,000 less than an After-Hours Manager. To make up some of the shortfall, I worked full-time night shift plus an additional 12-hour night shifts per week at a private hospital to make up the salary deficit. As an After-Hours Manager, I had earned enough that we could easily afford the mortgage on our beautiful home, and our active social life. Then, we had money to burn. Not anymore. Every penny counted and I was exhausted.

The mantle of failure furled its terrible wings and started to close around me. Blackness, outside of the glamour I wore at work, became my world. This was my first ever experience with the prospect of failure, which is clearly something I do not deal well with. As a high achiever, while the suspensions of candidature took a good deal of the pressure off me, I hated the fact that I had become a weak individual who couldn't just focus on the job at hand and get it done. After the second suspension of candidature, the months just flew by.

Academic degrees have time limitations for completion, and that time was rapidly descending upon me. This was a time for me to face up to the prospect of either recommencing the research or withdraw and just walk away, which was unthinkable, I have never walked away from anything in my life. I rang and spoke to my supervisor, Associate Professor Jeanne Madison, who is an amazing American-born woman. She has a vitality that is as infectious as is her intelligence and commonsense. I could always rely and trust in her for a frank, honest opinion. She is as honest as the day is long so I knew her answers would be truthful.

I explained to her the reasons for my call, what had happened and how I continued to struggle. I guess she was expecting to hear me say, "I am withdrawing from the degree". Rather than empathise with me that my life sucked, she gave me the kick in the arse that I needed and said in her wonderful American accent, "Oh for crying out loud Kathrine! Just write the damn thing!"

So, I did. I will be forever grateful to her. She is my hero.

I worked, came home, obsessed, smoked and drank. Alcohol was my temporary calming balm and I took to it like a lion to a fresh kill. I discovered if I didn't drink enough, I wouldn't be able to sleep and when I did, my dreams were a succession of nightmares. I would wake up in a sweat, panicked, not knowing what to do. Logic was unlikely to come from an alcohol-soaked brain. I was so tired of being sick and tired. But like all people who drink too much, I realised it was necessary to keep my drinking a secret, to ensure no one would ever guess that alcohol was a serious problem in my life. Every day, I looked forward to oblivion. For just a few short hours, I would be happy again. I would laugh and enjoy myself. I became aware of a significant change in my personality from the moment I took that first sip. I am certain no one in my family noticed my drinking problem. Eventually, my daughter expressed her concern but everyone else said nothing.

Each day, reality would return with the rise of the sun. I learned to hate the sunrise.

Not long after the news concerning the Intensive Care patient went live on air and in the newspapers, I was contacted by the Homicide police. They wanted to take a statement. Had this matter been dealt with as per the usual manner of Coronial Inquiries, this interview would have taken place years earlier, immediately following the death of the patient. The interview felt to me like another box ticking exercise. The issue was a political hot potato, there could be no apparent stone left unturned. I gave my statement to the two detectives who sat on the other side of my kitchen bench, both looking bored and disbelieving but I didn't give a damn about their opinions. I knew my interview would probably end up as shredded paper on the bottom of some child's mouse cage.

In total there were six nurses, including myself, who all had serious concerns about adverse patient outcomes and preventable patient deaths in the various hospitals where we worked. Narissa, the instigator, collected versions of the experiences of Meadhbh and Yanaha, the Operating Theatre Clinical Nurse Specialists and Violet who was an Intensive Care registered nurse. These three nurses worked at the same hospital. Simone was an endorsed enrolled nurse who worked at a neighbouring hospital, and I had been an After-Hours Manager at the Hospital from Hell.

Narissa, who had initially brought us all together, arranged a meeting on the 5th of November 2002 to meet with Craig Knowles, the (then) Minister for Health. She invited Meadhbh, Yanaha, Violet and Simone to accompany her to discuss their patient care concerns. I am perplexed to this day as to why she didn't invite me to attend this meeting, although I assume it was because I had showed her up on air. Narissa had her own agenda against the management of her employing hospital and exposed a series of highly publicised allegations to the effect that senior officers from within a NSW Area Health Service deliberately covered-up improper practices and adverse incidents by destroying or concealing relevant evidence after they had received complaints about such practices and incidents.

12

I lived day to day, working as many shifts as I could get. Employment guaranteed the money kept coming in and kept my alcohol consumption down. No professional nurse would ever consume alcohol before going on shift and I have never been one to drink after night shift. Being a person who needs order and loves straight lines, the thought of alcohol at breakfast time is simply illogical — my days off duty, however, were another story.

Life consisted of work/home, work/home, an endless loupe autopilot. I deliberately avoided the news and talking about the events of the past so I had no idea of the breadth of the investigations going on that erupted because of Narissa's claims about adverse patient outcomes. Even though she was the only nurse to actually seek media attention and speak out, public confidence in the NSW public health system plummeted. The meeting with the Minister for Health was the tip of the iceberg for what was to follow. Narissa, Meadhbh, Violet, Yanaha and Simone, because of their attendance at the meeting, were required to give evidence before the Legislative Council General Purpose Standing Committee inquiry into complaints handling within NSW Health. Imagine my surprise when I was notified that I was also required to attend.

One of the many positives of this level of Inquiry was, that deficits were identified and improved processes were put in place. This was the beginning of true clinical governance in Health in the state of New South Wales. It was because of our truths as nurses, albeit labelled as whistleblowers, that substandard quality and safety measures, adverse patient outcomes and major systems deficiencies were brought to the attention of the Australian public. There was a huge public display as heads rolled from on high. NSW Health had gotten rid of the bad eggs and had saved face. Or had they?

To this day, I don't know if at the time the information I reported as given to me by Monique, was ever declared to NSW Health. It was only after Narissa voiced the incident on public radio that the information was considered a sentinel event by the Hospital from Hell and NSW Health. Narissa was instrumental in all six of us being labelled as whistleblower nurses. She publicly advocated against poor patient outcomes and unexpected patient deaths occurring within her own employing hospital and deliberately contacted each of us for information about our own patient care concerns. At no time was I aware she intended to relay my experience to the media without first seeking my advice or consent. The consequence of the unauthorised release of all of the details of events previously discussed with Narissa was that the media concluded that we were a group of whistleblower nurses. This assumption progressed to misrepresentation and sensationalisation of the facts pertaining to each of the events as understood by myself and my colleagues. Because of Narissa's eagerness to communicate and cooperate with the media, she allowed herself to be erroneously portrayed as the chief of a group of vigilante whistleblower nurses — a title she did nothing to deny.

Narissa was obsessed by concern for patients, to the point where she made exaggerated statements like, "there have been hundreds of deaths!" No one stopped to say, "hang on, how can these nurses be whistleblowers if Narissa is the only one who actually spoke to the media?" It was gleeful guilt by association and the media had a field day. My colleagues and I spoke out because of expected professional conduct, good faith, beneficence, moral responsibility and the Australian cultural ethic 'to do the right thing'. We all reported through the established hierarchical channels of our individual employers. We were all professional advocates for patients. The label of whistleblower may have been sensational but could not have been further from the truth. We were front page news. We were media gold and we were fools.

In December 2003, Bret Walker SC was appointed Special Commissioner by the Letters Patent issued under the Special Commissions of Inquiry Act, 1983 [Act No.90, 1983] to inquire into and report on allegations of unsafe or inadequate patient care at two NSW hospitals. The first report released by The Inquiry was in March 2004, that recommended the conduct of twelve medical practitioners be investigated by the Health Care Complaints Commission (HCCC) and a further five practitioners be referred by the HCCC to the Medical Board.

The second Interim Report was issued on 1st June 2004 whereby the Commissioner recommended the doctors and nurses identified in a confidential report be investigated or have their performance assessed. On 30th July 2004, in addition to 17 suggestions for legislative change, the Commissioner made five recommendations regarding the methodology for analysis of the investigation into complaints and the availability of the findings created from such analysis and investigation.

These were tough times. Thanks to the media, our faces often appeared in the nightly news and on current affairs programs. I would turn up for my agency shifts, which were always night duty; firstly, because the night shift attracts a higher penalty rate and secondly so I could keep my head down and maintain a low profile. Even with the reduced staff numbers on night shift, invariably someone would say, "I know you from somewhere. Oh, I know! You were on A Current Affair with Ray Martin."

He was a long-time host of A Current Affair and to this day is considered one of Australia's best journalists. I found him to be ethical and honest and an all-round lovely, genuine man. He came to my house with his television crew to interview me and his empathy was palpable. He was supportive of us. Apart from Narissa, we were never known by our names. We were always referred to as 'the whistleblower nurses from Camden and Campbelltown'. He was empathetic and said he believed we had all done the right thing by exposing adverse patient outcomes and poor practice standards. He tried to run the television interview a second time but it was shut down. Politics before truth, every time.

In 2004, after working many shifts in maternity, the acting position of Nursing Unit Manager Level 3 was advertised. There had been an acting Nursing Unit Manager of Ward X for quite some time, she was well-liked and skilled so, in truth, based on my track record to date, I wasn't hopeful, but I applied for the job regardless. I was contacted by the (then) Senior Nurse Manager of the maternity service. She was surprisingly candid about what the role would entail and didn't sugar coat anything. What the service was looking to recruit as a matter of urgency was a change agent, not simply a manager of a maternity ward.

I had significant experience with the management of change within nursing. This job sounded like it had my name on it. The mandate was huge and involved the overall responsibility for antenatal and postnatal services and the Midwifery at Home program — where midwives visit women at home to support them with breast feeding and baby care. The person for this job had to have the experience and the drive to facilitate positive change as the services involved had considerable challenges in terms of skill mix, skill level and willingness to accept change.

The mandate was a huge ask for one person to undertake. From experience I knew this organisation to be troubled in terms of reputation and staff retention. It also had an entrenched reputation for bullying and harassment.

I didn't even think about it. I applied for the job, and I was offered an interview! The sense of relief was overwhelming. I felt as though finally there was light at the end of the tunnel. This job came with a good salary. If I was successful, there would be no more worrying about shifts, or the lack thereof. A permanent position (albeit acting) came with holidays, paid sick leave and long service leave; the dark days would be behind me. This was the chance I had prayed for. Shortly after the interview, I was advised I was the successful candidate. I accepted the offer.

I focussed on getting my career back on track while trying to leave the horror of the past behind me. As an agency nurse, I had worked many shifts in Maternity, so I knew a good number of the staff. I also knew the politics within the department. Was I so desperate to secure a permanent position that my brain, out of desperation, obliterated what I already knew to be true? I was Daniel. And I was walking into the lions' den.

13

Shortly after commencing employment, I was summoned to the Director of Nursing's office (something that always makes me nervous). An invitation to her office always came with an agenda. I had met this woman before. She sat on the interview panel for the After-Hours Manager's job I successfully interviewed for at the hospital where I was originally employed as the Delivery Suite Manager. She had a reputation for being fair and was known to be a strong advocate for nursing.

We chatted for a while and she made it quite clear she knew 'who I was' in terms of speaking out and being labelled as a whistleblower. She also made no bones about the fact that she had endorsed my appointment because she supported the stand that my five colleagues and I had taken.

I started to relax when suddenly she paused and glared at me. Jesus! My heart stopped. I will never forget the next 60 seconds of our conversation for as long as I live. Candidly, she asked, "Would you ever blow the whistle on us here at Hospital X?"

I met her stare and responded, "If a patient is murdered or comes to harm because of poor practice or adverse care, and the management of this organisation does nothing about it, then, yes, every time, yes!"

She nodded and smiled. "Good enough".

I soon discovered the job was as sticky as a spider's web. The role presented a tricky, professional conundrum when I discovered that professional practice was at the heart of the issues for this service. The definition of a midwife, according to the Nurses and Midwives Board of Australia: 'The midwife is recognised as a responsible and accountable professional who works in partnership with women to give the necessary support, care and advice during pregnancy, labour and the postpartum period, to conduct birth as the midwife's own responsibility and to provide care for the newborn'. To address the clinical deficits for a considerable number of staff members and the professional issues for this service, the mandates for my role as the newly appointed Nursing Unit Manager Level 3 blew out like sails on a Spanish Galleon.

The mandate for this role:

- Development of a Model of Care for Ward X - As per a report from a formal Consultancy firm employed to address the chronic workforce issues between these two wards.

- Address of the issues of skill mix, by planning, integrating and evaluating the clinical up-skilling of endorsed enrolled nurses, to in part, address the current shortage of Registered Midwives.

- Facilitation of up-skilling of endorsed enrolled nurses by enrolment in and successful completion of the Level 2 Neonatal Course to participate in care of Level 2 neonates.

- Creation and promotion of a 'one ward' philosophy to combine the two 54 bed wards.

- Conduct a service review for the Domiciliary Midwifery Program with recommendations for succession planning.

- Conduct a service review for the Foetal Maternal Assessment Unit with recommendations for improving efficiency, service promotion and succession planning.

- Quantification of the clinical challenges applicable to staff, who, for many years, had not worked outside of their present clinical area.

- Design, implement and evaluate a systematic rotation of all staff across the antenatal and postnatal clinical areas, to ensure all staff are clinically competent.

- Address roster challenges with a mandate to promote fairness and equity of opportunity with rosters for all staff
- Quantification and address bullying and harassment across Wards Y and X and to promote and implement the 'Zero Tolerance Policy'.
- Facilitation of productive workflows in nursing teams
- Review of the Domiciliary Midwifery Service to promote efficiency and marketing of the service to the patients of Wards Y and X, as a patient flow strategy and to create a culture of normalising birth with early return of women to the home environment, supported by home visit midwives.
- Plan, develop and implement the establishment of a neonatal 4 bed Level 2 nursery on Ward Y.
- Plan, develop and evaluate a neonatal education accreditation program, in consultation with the Neonatal Nurse Educator, for Midwives and Endorsed Enrolled Nurses to staff the Level 2 nursery of Ward Y.
- Plan and develop in consultation with Clinical Nurse Consultant of Paediatrics and Director of Paediatrics, policies and procedures to underpin neonatal care that is consistent with practice in the Neonatal Intensive Care Unit.
- Identify and address existing WH&S issues for Wards Y and X.

It was clear to me from the scope of this role, that the mandate was destined to fail from the outset. This environment was like living in a perpetual storm, where a maelstrom of issues had been allowed to fester which impacted directly upon job satisfaction, patient safety and patient outcomes.

The Antenatal and Postnatal Wards traditionally had been very separate entities in terms of clinical service provision, staffing and attitudes. There was palpable angst between these two areas, which my observations led me to believe was firmly rooted in professional frustration. If the Antenatal Ward required additional staff, the vast majority of the postnatal staff, because of workforce stagnation, were not skilled in antenatal care and therefore were not confident or competent to be responsible for a full Antenatal patient load. A good many of these midwives were terrified of being deployed to the Antenatal Ward and were never deployed to the Delivery Suite. To me, it was obvious. The hostility and animosity that the staff displayed towards each other was due to being deskilled clinically and feeling threatened by the potential that they could be deployed to another area that was clearly not only out of their comfort zone, but outside of their scope of practice. This was one of the facts that fuelled this toxic work environment. I always found it sad when the midwives belittled each other about skill levels when in reality, the blame lay with the organisation. The responsibility to ensure currency of skills is a managerial responsibility. These staff were the victims of poor leadership, faulty service structure and no succession planning, which resulted in non-alpha individuals struggling to survive in this very hostile environment. It was wrong that the problems that existed between these two wards were attributed to the staff, when the blame fairly and squarely should have been laid at the feet of the leaders of the Division and the executive management.

Professional jealously also played a significant part in the grumbling animosity between these two wards. The staffing of the 30-bed Postnatal Ward was almost double that of the 24- bed Antenatal Ward which to the reasonable person is understandable, given the rapid turnaround time, the high caesarean section rate, the additional six beds and of course the additional care factor for the babies. Yet, the inability of a good number of postnatal midwives to step up clinically, was a bug bear for the antenatal staff. If an additional postnatal staff member was required on the postnatal ward, an antenatal staff member could be relied upon to take on a full unsupervised patient load. However, a frustration for the antenatal midwives was that it was always a member of the antenatal staff who was deployed if the Delivery Suite was overwhelmed (which often was). Years of static work practice meant some of the postnatal staff hadn't worked in Delivery Suite for years — some hadn't done so since the completion of their training. In my view, this was an self-created organisational problem.

There was no ceiling on the number of women who could choose to deliver at this hospital. The numbers of women booked for confinement more than breached the amount of available bedspace and staff. Yet the 'open bookings' policy persisted — despite protestations and clear evidence that demand well and truly, exceeded capacity. This situation was to the detriment of patient care and exacerbated already strained relationships between the staff. This organisation had a particularly negative reputation in terms of being a tough place to work which negatively impacted upon recruitment and retention of midwives.

Prior to my appointment as the manager, I was aware there was a serious and entrenched problem with bullying and harassment and that these behaviours were generated primarily by one of the Maternity managers. Nursing socialisation was a powerful thing, akin to pack mentality. If a nurse wanted to be accepted and not bullied, the nurse had to emulate the behaviours of the more senior nurses in order to be offered a safe place within the nursing hierarchy. Regardless of whether the senior nurse was a bully or a nurturer, the beta members of the pack had to emulate those behaviours which were akin to alpha/beta pack behaviour. Mirroring of alpha behaviour resulted in acceptance into the wider nursing social circle and sanctuary under a senior nurse's wing to be mentored, supervised and out of the firing line. Bullying was a daily fact of life between these two wards and is a challenge for the profession as a whole.

The most significant bullying appeared to be generated by one ward and after a very expensive review by a private company, a report was tabled and the Nursing Unit Manager of that ward was removed from the position. The staff by now, were very jaded and had been affected badly by the screaming, unprofessional, demeaning manager. My challenge was to identify the players and work with the staff to encourage improvement in the way they communicated to each other and to build trusting relationships and tolerance. Sounds simple enough, right?

Nursing is a 24/7 service. When I was a junior nurse, like everyone else, I took the good with the bad. If I were rostered for four days off that included a weekend, it was like winning the lottery. If my name was against the line with four weeks straight of night duty — too bad, someone had to do it. Not so in this day of modern nursing. The trend for nurses today is that part time work is preferred to full time. Also, shift work and weekend work are not part of a long-term plan for a career in nursing. In short, the expectations of being a nurse now are vastly different than when I entered the profession in 1978.

Cronyism was alive and well in the hospital I was working. On Ward Y, as part of the reward system offered by the newly deposed manager, the chosen were given set shifts, which meant they worked the shifts they wanted, and it was set in stone. If roster changes were required to meet workload demands or to cover sick leave, the chosen were never considered as part of the solution to the staffing deficit. I met with the staff and explained the inequity of this practice and that fairness in rostering practice would now come into play.

This proposed change caused an absolute uproar and sick leave skyrocketed. In an attempt to foster the concept of fair play, I implemented a pro rata limit on the number of shift requests a staff member could make on a roster. The algorithm was based on the number of hours that were worked. I mean really, for a full-time staff member to have twenty-eight requested shifts for a monthly roster is hardly equitable. There was much grumbling, however, for a while, those who were never rostered off for a weekend got to spend time with their families and those who now worked the occasional weekend sharpened their knives to stab me in the back. As is the way of things, the bullies on the ward soon intimidated the less powerful into making roster swap requests. Before I knew it, the roster, based on the request system, had virtually reverted to its original form.

Intimidation is a powerful tool. I had already realised this was a battle I was not going to win. This situation just didn't sit well with me. Fair play was required for all of the staff who never got a weekend off and who worked more than their share of night duty. I delegated responsibility of the roster to one of the chosen. If that midwife was deemed responsible for the roster, fairness had to come into play unless he/she wanted to be criticised and accused of cronyism. This action didn't solve the problem completely, but the roster became more equitable.

I have always been the kind of person with an absolute need to understand the 'why' of things. I do not engage in tasks just because that is how it has always been done. I am not good at being given orders unless I understand the purpose of the request, that it makes sense and that it serves a positive purpose. I would have made a terrible soldier.

My experience as an agency nurse who had worked many shifts on Ward Y, ensured I was well aware of the 'bedside surveillance' approach to monitoring babies that required extra observation or care. I was also aware that, on many occasions, the observations were missed, sometimes for hours in succession, due to the pace of the midwifery patient load on the ward. When I worked on this ward, I found the staff to be experienced, collegial and very hard working. However, it was obvious to anyone who gave a damn that the staffing and the skill mix was simply inadequate to offer these babies the care they needed, and the policies demanded. Added to this issue, there was insufficient space in the Neonatal Intensive Care Unit to accept these babies to ensure they were appropriately monitored. These were two reasons for lack of neonatal surveillance on Ward Y. Both reasons were legitimate and were beyond the control of the staff. On a number of occasions, I observed another reason that put these babies at risk and it was attitudinal. The Neonatal nursing staff didn't accept that babies who required intravenous antibiotics, blue light phototherapy or blood sugar monitoring were candidates to utilise their expensive resources by being housed in a Neonatal Intensive Care Unit. Neonatal nurses are a clear and distinct, very separate breed from midwives and they clash frequently. To be a neonatal nurse, a midwifery qualification is not required.

Patients in Neonatal Intensive Care are likely to be ventilated and very often critical. This 'value laden' conundrum resulted in friction between the neonatal nurses and the midwives of Ward Y, the result of which ended in declarations of incompetence, eye rolling or the favourite of all favourite nursing put-downs, "Oh you want to send the baby down here, (to Neonatal Intensive Care) because you can't cope?"

Without fail, the put downs were deliberate and intentionally personal. There was never any acknowledgement of how hard these postnatal nurses/midwives worked because the neonatal staff did not work there.

The stark reality was that adverse outcomes of high acuity babies being cared for at the mother's bedside did occur on Ward Y. These outcomes didn't occur because of incompetence or from a lack of caring. It came down to the fact that this ward was resource poor in terms of staff numbers and lacked an appropriate environment where these babies could be under constant supervision. Extreme pressure was brought to bear on the midwives in charge of these unwell babies. Their workload, from my observation, was beyond unreasonable. If any of the vital sign observations were noted to have been missed, an incident report was submitted, and the midwife was required to explain why he or she was delinquent in their care. Never was there any degree of responsibility accepted by the management that the workload was just beyond human capacity.

I don't condone documentation of 'radar observations'—ever. But I do understand why in this situation this phenomenon occurred. If there was a change in the baby's condition overnight, the nurses/midwives to my knowledge and to the best of his/her ability, would observe the baby or if concerned the mother would raise the alarm. A paediatric medical officer would be called to review the baby. If the baby was well and no alarms were raised during the night, just before change of shift, I had witnessed hours of observations documented, all within normal, acceptable ranges. This way, the outgoing midwife didn't get her arse kicked for not having ten arms and five extra hours in the shift. However unrealistic, expectation often resulted in creative solutions.

> None are so blind as those who do not see.
>
> Mathew 9:26-27

As a 'dinosaur' nurse, I have, throughout my career, worked with endorsed and non-endorsed enrolled nurses. I hold great respect for the role. In my opinion these are the nurses who often make a real difference to a patient's hospital experience. They make the time to wash a patient's hair or ensure that pressure care is done on time. I have friends who are endorsed enrolled nurses and I admire them immensely. A good too many registered nurses in my experience suffer with 'the white shoe' syndrome which equates to exclusive involvement in important matters such as accompanying medical officers on 'medical officers' rounds' or administering medications. Patient care such as hair washing, toenail cutting or wiping someone's bum are clearly deemed to be roles for someone less important than them. I loathe registered nurses who behave like this.

Recruitment and retention of midwives is a world-wide problem. Demand well and truly exceeds supply. Yet the patients kept coming and they still need care. I had an idea. To bridge the gap and decrease the staffing/skill deficit, I proposed an advanced scope of practice for endorsed enrolled nurses. The theory behind this proposal was to up-skill the endorsed enrolled nurses, which in turn would free up the midwives to have more time to spend with the women and attend procedures such as postnatal checks, tricky breast-feeding situations, and management of obstetric emergencies such as post-partum haemorrhage, which are all strictly in the domain of a registered midwife. This proposal went down like a lead balloon with the midwives. The endorsed enrolled nurses saw the proposition for what it was—an opportunity! The midwives bitched about midwifery care being the domain of the midwife and that endorsed enrolled nurses had no place working in maternity, yet no better suggestions were forthcoming about how to better utilise the time and skills of the scarce midwives. It was obvious that my decision was not going to win me any friends. The solution was to delegate those facets of nursing care that did not necessarily require the skills of a midwife to the endorsed enrolled nurses and free up the midwives to do that for which they are professionally accountable. To some of the midwives, I became public enemy number one.

I collected reams of data in the first few months after my appointment. The factors that impacted upon this very troubled ward soon became obvious and were quantifiable. Firstly, profound elitist midwife behaviour was rife, secondly, rejection of endorsed enrolled nurses working on their turf and probably most importantly, completely unrealistic expectations on the part of management. Based on my previous knowledge, from having worked on this ward as a midwife, I focused on what I considered to be the ward's top priority—keeping the babies safe.

I quantified the number and type of adverse neonatal outcomes that had occurred on the ward in the previous 12 months. It was no surprise to me that the numbers were significant. It was this information that confirmed the need to change the current practice of bedside observation of babies. The data also provided a scope of education and training for midwives and endorsed enrolled nurses. This data could not be ignored. After all, if what I had discovered was not taken seriously by management and a baby incurred an adverse outcome, they feared I would go to the media. After all, apparently, I was a whistleblower nurse.

After the data I collected was circulated, it was agreed that there needed to be a better option for observing babies who required extra care. I was assigned the responsibility of converting a room in the middle of the ward into a four bed Level 2 nursery. A highly collegial working party was formed that included me, the Director of Paediatrics and Clinical Nurse Consultants from both Neonatal Intensive Care and Paediatrics. We worked at a furious pace to define a scope of service, algorithms and policies and procedures, all of which were written and signed off. The scope of practice for the Level 2 nursery included jaundiced babies who required phototherapy; preterm babies — greater than 36 weeks gestation; babies of diabetic mothers; or any baby that required more frequent than 4-hourly observations would receive the care and observations they required by an appropriately trained staff member in the dedicated Level 2 nursery. Ironically, if the Level 2 nursery was full, any overflow babies would be accepted into Neonatal Intensive Care — no questions asked. I will forever be proud of that achievement.

The observation and resource issue related to care of these babies was solved. Level 2 babies were cared for in the nursery by competent staff, which presented the next thorny issue. To staff the nursery, a midwife who would normally have been part of the ward team was required to be rostered to the nursery. While some of the midwives were keen to work in the nursery for a break from the hectic pace of the ward, others were not. I needed a plan. We had all worked too hard for this to fail now.

There were a number of skilled endorsed enrolled nurses employed on Ward Y. Their practice was very limited when it came to midwifery care. Basically, they could do observations and basic clinical work, but the midwifery component of responsibility such as breast feeding and postnatal care was definitely well and truly in the domain of the midwives, the supposed experts.

In 1987, I disproved the expert theory. At 29, I had been a practicing midwife for 8 years when N. was born. After birthing and learning how to breast feed, I wanted to run out and apologise to every woman I had ever cared for. Prior to becoming a mother, I thought I understood birthing and those early months of motherhood. I completely underestimated just how incredibly painful and gruelling labour and birthing can be. The same applied to breast feeding which of course is natural— a natural source of food for the baby, that is. There is nothing natural or innate about breast feeding when it comes to knowing how to go about it. Breast feeding is a technique that is learned. Again, I offer my most sincere apologies to all of those women who were the victims of my spruiking as a non-experienced breast feeder. Breast feeding, like parenting, is a skill that is acquired over time. I had helped hundreds of women to breast feed, but when it came to me, I had absolutely no clue. As they say, it is harder than it looks. My husband and I still laugh about when he came to visit on the second night after I had given birth. In all seriousness I said to him, "Be careful where you walk. If you see anything brown and shrivelled up on the floor, for God's sake don't walk on them; that will be my bloody nipples, because they will have fallen off!"

This experience taught me a huge lesson. Personal experience of birthing, breast feeding and mothering is the best teacher. I was a stellar 'textbook' midwife, but the reality of what I experienced was never expressed in any of the books that I studied. I now know the advice I offered my past patients was less than realistic. This experience affirmed that just because I was a midwife, I was not an expert.

The blatant and highly offensive view held by some of the midwives that there was no place for endorsed enrolled nurses in midwifery was a miasma that was a constant, undermining presence. Yet, a good number of the endorsed enrolled nurses that worked on Ward Y were mothers with years of experience — valuable experience that could have benefited new mothers who struggled with breast feeding and baby care. They could have certainly offered better advice than I had before having my first child. In truth, the role delineation came down to professional territorialism. Engagement of endorsed enrolled nurses in the realm of breast feeding and postnatal care was perceived by some midwives to be in clear conflict with the ethos of care that had traditionally been provided by them and them alone. The seed of unpopularity was planted but, to make the Level 2 nursery a functional success, again, I needed a plan — and fast! This was when I started to consider a role for endorsed enrolled nurses in the newly established Level 2 nursery.

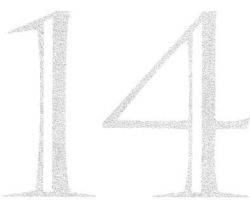

I am now and forever more proud to be a midwife. I am not however proud of the elitist views of a good many of my colleagues that non-midwives are persona non grata when it comes to midwifery care. The harsh reality is that there are not enough midwives in the workforce and as the population continues to increase and midwives age, there needs to be creative solutions put in place to ensure midwives are present at birthing, are champions for breast feeding and continue to provide women-centred care.

Howls of professional fury will be heard nation-wide regarding my next statement but, this is my memoir and therefore my reality. I have never believed a midwife is required for standard postnatal care — most women are essentially well and go home soon after birth. Of course, if there are complications such as postpartum haemorrhage then a midwife is required to attend to the patient as this is a potentially life-threatening situation. I also do not believe the care of the newborn is requiring of the skills of a midwife. For years, Neonatal Intensive Care Units have employed registered nurses with stand-alone qualifications. They have also employed endorsed enrolled nurses who, through education, supervision and mentorship, have become very skilled in the care of unwell babies.

The idea of an advanced model of care for enrolled nurses, although part of my employment mandate, was from the outset met with professional opposition and hostility from some of the senior midwives who openly campaigned for enrolled nurses to be expelled from maternity all together.

This was another conundrum. The service had babies that required higher levels of nursing surveillance. The newly commissioned Level 2 nursery was ready to go but where was the human resource plan? I realised in trepidation, the only real solution to the staffing issue for the nursery was obvious.

I am an idealistic fool. Buoyed by a solution to the staffing issue and after a discussion with my manager that this was legally and professionally acceptable but most importantly doable, I issued an Expression of Interest to all of the endorsed enrolled nurses to work in the nursery. Education was paramount. Once those who had taken up the offer had successfully completed the Level 2 Nursery certification program underwent a period of clinical supervision and competency sign off. At that point, they were ready to fly solo and staff the new Level 2 ward nursery. I thought this to be a stroke of brilliance.

A good number of the endorsed enrolled nurses jumped at the chance to gain new skills and be valued for the care they offered the babies. To a select few of the senior midwives, I was Judas. The knives were out, as were the poisoned pens. The Director of Nursing received anonymous letters advising I had deliberately and knowingly put babies at risk by the advancement of endorsed enrolled nurse practice. Numerous times I was summoned to the Director of Nursing's office to answer to these allegations — which were just that, allegations made by elitist midwives who did not want the status quo of mother / baby midwifery care interfered with, or changed from how it had been delivered for millennia.

It is ironic, during the Medieval Inquisitions, midwives were persecuted, accused and 'tried' as witches for offering care to the sick, and were burned at the stake. I was offside with the senior midwife power players. They rejected out of hand any increase in endorsed enrolled nurse practice and responsibility. This select group of midwives were determined to see me crucified in order to resume the status quo — their status quo. It was after an anonymous missive was delivered to the Minister for Health that the senior managers who recruited me to implement these changes, started stepping back as they relinquished their support for the plan they agreed to and turned their backs on me. When the Minister for Health was notified about anything regarding professional practice in a specific hospital, regardless of whether the allegations were truth, lie or dare, the organisation would back down like a well-trained dog and behave. This action by the midwives was a lay-down Misère play, orchestrated to get rid of me and the alleged threat I posed to midwifery practice.

The Director of Nursing was empathetic; she was well aware of the enormity of the problems in this maternity unit. She also realised, given my past, the toll all of this was having on me. We believed we knew who the coward was who wrote to the Minister of Health as the language used in the letters was constant and clearly from the same person. The same person who felt so strongly about the risks I allegedly posed not only to the babies but also to the profession, had the strength of conviction but not the guts to sign the letters. It didn't even matter. The desired purpose had been achieved — the damage was done. I continued in the role but was stone-walled at every turn.

To this day, I do not understand how the benefit of endorsed enrolled nurses working in the nursery to free up midwives to spend more time with the women was obvious only to me. The endorsed enrolled nurses continued to work in the Level 2 nursery which was a huge success. But by then, I had so many knives in my back that I was stymied and ineffective as a leader. Is it any wonder I loathe cowards.

This was an exhausting job, not only because of the constant tension regarding the endorsed enrolled nurses working in the

Level 2 nursery, but because of the many extracurricular hours I put in at home. I researched endlessly, trying to find a solution that would promote improved relationships between Ward Y and Ward X while heading off the white ants who continued to sabotage any form of change. I understand change is associated with resistance — humans like stability, they need stability. Change invokes feelings of loss of control and vulnerability. It was an uphill battle.

After a year of banging my head against a brick wall to try and invoke positive change, a relieving After-Hours Manager's position was advertised. As I read the advertisement, I experienced an overwhelming sense of déjà vu, but I applied anyway. I was bone tired. The Nursing Unit Manager Level 3 job was incredibly demanding. If I could work a shift or two a week as an After-Hours Manger, that would give me the respite I needed to regain the energy to push on with the mandates of my substantive position. I was offered an interview — another rush of déjà vu. The Director of Nursing was the convener of the panel. It was a surreal moment, like being sucked into a vortex, back in time, 20 years prior when she had been on the interview panel for the After-Hours Manager's role at the hospital where I was the Delivery Suite Manager. The interview went well and I was hopeful.

A few days later, the Director of Nursing requested I come to her office. Excitement made my heart pound. Was she was calling me to congratulate me on my application and that I had been appointed as a relieving After-Hours Manager? I felt a ton of weight lift from my shoulders. This job would give me the break I needed to carry on the good fight and push on with the directives of my substantive role to improve the maternity services offered by Ward X and Ward Y. It would be good to be back in the after-hours environment where anything and everything can and usually does happen. It is a job for those who can think on their feet.

I arrived in Nursing Administration and advised the receptionist who I was and that the Director of Nursing had requested I meet with her. She picked up the phone and said a few quiet words. The Director of Nursing opened the door and invited me in. I was smiling so wide with excitement, my face almost cracked. She started the discussion with praise for my achievements so far. Oh no. In my experience, a poor outcome is always preceded by a positive wind-up. A sinking feeling began to form in my belly when I realised what was happening — the old KKK principle — Kiss, Kick, Kiss.

The Director of Nursing sighed and her shoulders drooped. "I called you here today to advise you were the successful applicant for the role of relieving After-Hours Manager."

Yes! Big smile back in place. (Kiss) Odd... Her sad demeanour didn't change. She put both of her hands out in front of her, palms upward on the desk. "I am so sorry. You were by far the best applicant for the job, but I can't offer the role to you. The General Manager has been informed by New South Wales Health that you have a lifetime ban on career advancement, for your participation in the 'whistleblower' fallout from Camden and Campbelltown" (Kick).

She then leaned forward, touched my hand and congratulated me on the improvements I had achieved thus far in my current role (Kiss). I was stunned. Suddenly, there was no air in the room. I was suffocating as panic rose up in my chest like a tsunami. I couldn't speak. I was like an automaton. I stood, turned my back on the Director of Nursing, opened the door, went back to my office, picked up my handbag and went home. Fuck!

The attention of the Minister for Health generated a time of great flux for the maternity service at this hospital. There was to be an area position formally created — yet another tier of management for the maternity services. The current Acting Area Senior Nurse Manager of the service was a very professional, empathetic and well-respected midwife. In my view, she was a shoo-in for the promotion. It is a good thing I didn't bet on the outcome.

The position I was recruited for was an 'acting' position which means the position is defined for a specified period of time or until the person has outlived their usefulness and needs to be gone. This generally happens when there is an extensive period of leave to be replaced, or as in my case, the position was created in an attempt to try and solve the myriad of problems within the organisation's maternity unit. I do believe that in the beginning, all of the senior managers were committed to the mandates as defined to me and wanted the problems solved. I also know that when the going got tough i.e. letters to the Minister for Health, the management's level of commitment shrivelled up and died. The bully girls had woven their magic and very successfully undermined me and the mandates I had been given. They had won.

After all of my hard spent effort, the senior managers caved and the two wards went back to being two separate entities with a Nursing Unit Manager to be appointed to each area. My position, the Level 3, was to be abolished. The Senior Nurse Manager of the division explained the decision to me, which in essence, was that the issues regarding these two wards was a political hot potato and was now firmly planted in the too hard basket. No one had the balls to push on. I was informed if I applied for either of the two Nursing Unit Manager jobs, I would be appointed to the role of Nursing Unit Manager of the Postnatal Ward. The role of the manager of the Antenatal Ward was to be given to the person who had been acting in the role for some time. She had much less experience than me, no tertiary qualifications and no management track record to speak of. But she was a good employee who did what she was told, didn't question decisions and didn't rock the boat. When the job was advertised, even though postnatal midwifery is not my passion, it was a permanent position, so I applied for the job. I didn't want to be out in the cold again.

After the applications closed, I was invited to interview and to be truthful, I was feeling pretty confident, although my nose was out of joint that I didn't have the opportunity to apply for the antenatal position. The Senior Nurse Manager phoned me and asked me to meet with her in her office. Yes! She was calling to tell me I was the successful applicant for a job I didn't really want, but a job is a job.

I had a lot of respect for this woman. She was very fair and had a good understanding of the issues that plagued the maternity unit. We chatted for a bit and out of the blue she said, "You didn't get the job." She sighed and said, "You're not the only one. I didn't get the job either."

I was dumbstruck. Who could have interviewed for the position that had more experience than me? The power players had won. The person who was appointed to the role had no previous management experience, was a newbie in terms of postgraduate experience and was malleable to the demands of the senior midwives who would either make her or break her. The latter was the eventual outcome.

I, like the Senior Nurse Manager, was out of a job, but now I was faced with a future that precluded any appointment to management roles, as per the ban imposed by New South Wales Health. People who learn of this fact often said to me, "How could that possibly happen?"

My answer, "Equal opportunity employment principles are lip service, nothing more, nothing less."

In the eyes of New South Wales Health and the profession of nursing, I had committed a cardinal sin. By virtue of the information offered to me by Monique, I was perceived to have deliberately made the public aware of what was always supposed to have been kept 'in-house'. I had been tried and found guilty without even being aware that this decision had ever been made. I was never formally notified or formally sanctioned. But as I have already said — nursing is a very small world.

The wolf was back clawing at the door and once again I frantically trawled through advertisements looking for a job. The ban against career advancement continually rattled around in my brain. I am a warrior, but this was a time in my life when I realised the truth in the saying, "you can't fight city hall".

I stopped looking for management roles, as that horse had clearly bolted. I rejected the thought of returning to agency work, I just could not be assigned to clinical situations that were beyond my scope of practice. It was 2006 and I had no time to be choosey. I had walked away from the Nursing Unit Manager Level 3 job with a few weeks of annual leave and that was it. I swallowed my pride and applied for a position as a midwife on the Antenatal ward at the same hospital that had just terminated my services.

Desperate times call for pride to be swallowed and desperate measures. The reasons for this decision were three-fold: the hospital involved the least amount of travelling to and from work; I was just too worn out to apply myself to learning another hospital's routines and start from the ground up as a newbie; and the third reason was perhaps the most important to me — I could work permanent night shift to keep my head down and make a reasonable wage by virtue of night shift and weekend penalty rates.

The Acting Nursing Unit Manager of the Antenatal Ward was now officially appointed to the role. She was a good midwife who cared about the women. We had become friends when I was in the position of Nursing Unit Manager Level 3. She had been employed at this organisation for a long time. Ironically, she interviewed me for the position of midwife on the Antenatal Ward. Of course, I was offered a job and she welcomed me back with open arms. After all, experienced midwives are as rare as hen's teeth.

15

The saying 'familiarity breeds contempt' was never truer than with the events that would impact my friendship with the Nursing Unit Manager of the Antenatal Ward. Staff would come to me for advice on clinical or professional issues. Now, I have no doubt that these conversations were relayed back to the Nursing Unit Manager by those who would be rewarded for being her eyes and ears. Over time, our relationship deteriorated. I began to lose respect for her as a manager and she, maybe because of professional jealousy or because of events to come, no doubt came to regret employing me. To this day, I am not certain if she passed me in the street whether she would give me more than an obligatory nod and keep walking.

I was dissatisfied professionally. I was angry that my career trajectory was stymied and that for the rest of my working life, as a clinician I would have little or no opportunity to review policy and procedures or invoke positive change in patient care. I held a Bachelor of Health Management and had no hope of ever utilising those skills. I am an out-of-the-box, global thinker, but also clearly gullible and naive. When I identified a situation or an issue that if undertaken differently, would result in an improved outcome, I would email the Nursing Unit Manager, as our hours of work didn't lend to us running into each other very often. I will never be sure whether she resented my input and interpreted such as interference in her domain, or whether the fact that I had been in a superior position was threatening to her. Either way, my suggestions fell on deaf ears. I stopped trying to strive for service improvement and concentrated on keeping my head down. I didn't want any trouble. I needed this job. Frustration was my constant companion

The high point in my life in 2006 was when I finished researching for the Master of Health Management [hons] degree. I then wrote the thesis and submitted the work. On the day I graduated, my family cheered from the audience and Associate Professor Jeanne Madison lit up like a beacon. She knew how hard it had been for me. Once a wise woman, always a wise woman. Unlike me, she realised I possessed the inner strength and fortitude to push on and finish the degree. On graduation day, when it was my turn to step up on the podium, I broke with protocol, blew a kiss to her where she sat with the other robed academics, then beat my fist across my heart three times.

It was a great moment. I was the first in the family with a master's degree.

I have always had a busy brain and boredom is my nemesis. With all of the study behind me, I needed a creative outlet, something that would occupy and enthuse me while continuing to go to work, doing what I had to do and keeping under the radar. Out of the blue, an idea struck me. It was like a revelation. I have always loved reading. Words are like music to me and I have always loved to write. I decided to write a book of fiction. I had no clue how to write a book, but I was pretty sure I could do it. It couldn't be that hard, right?

This was a life changing moment for me because I suddenly realised that when I was writing fiction, anything was possible and the story was only limited by my imagination. I also realised that my happy thoughts surround me when I was in the zone, creating characters and worlds. When I wrote, I left my life and immersed myself into the worlds of my creation. As with every other facet of my life, I had two speeds, either flat out or stopped, with nothing in-between. I became obsessed with the fiction I was writing. I have always loved the Scots and Scottish history, so I immersed myself in fiction that celebrated all things Scottish. It was at this point that I realised I had always been fascinated by paranormal and fantasy stories. So, it is no surprise that my story took a paranormal/fantasy turn. I worked on the manuscript slavishly and after 158,000 words it was finished. I had written a book! Now what?

Boredom once again raised its ugly head. The news was still full of discussions and recommendations from the Inquires into healthcare in New South Wales. I honestly tried to stay as far from that as I could get. It was just too hard to exist in a world where stories of grief and despair kept coming from the two hospitals under investigation. I needed a distraction.

I have always loved academic study. I had for some time, been aware of a sense of longing and emptiness rattling around in the back of my brain after I finished the Master of Health Management [hons]. In truth, the completion of the degree left a gaping hole in my life. The next thing I knew, I was talking to my hero, Associate Professor Jeanne Madison, from the University of New England. I wanted to undertake a PhD, but typical of me, I wanted to undertake a study like no other. I wanted to tell the story of the journey of the whistleblower nurses as a collective.

The outcomes of the Inquiries into healthcare were shocking and it was clear that New South Wales Health had real problems in terms of critical incident handling, reporting systems and governance processes to prevent those events from happening again. After discussing my experience of being labelled as a whistleblower and what I knew of the events that had led to the Inquiries, Jeanne's eyes lit up and she told me. I was sitting on research gold. I knew the other nurses by virtue of professional association. They had trusted me in the past and I hoped they would trust me again and be candid in the telling of their stories.

We had all been caught up in the nightmare of public exposure by two hospitals.

A PhD was exactly what I need to undertake, not only because it was a means of occupying my arse-numbingly bored-at-work brain, but I would get answers to the questions I had sought for years. Once the seed of thought about starting a PhD was planted, I really started to think hard about the other nurses who had been cited as 'whistleblowers'. What the hell had happened to them after they had unwittingly risked everything thanks to Narissa making their stories public? I had been severely sanctioned and punished by New South Wales Health. Had my colleagues suffered likewise?

I bit the bullet, enrolled and was accepted into a PhD program. My supervisors were (no surprises here) Associate Professor Jeanne Madison and Professor Victor Minichiello. I had some idea how to conduct and write up qualitative research as I had written a research-based thesis for the Master of Health Management [hons], for a PhD however, the bar was set up in the ether.

I was excited to be back in the land of academia. For the first time in a long time, I was truly happy. I regularly interacted with Jeanne Madison which in itself, provided jolts of re-energisation for me. Have you ever met a person who when they speak with connection and clarity, that suddenly everything is clear and understandable? She is one of those people.

I was at the beginning of the study; I really didn't know how or what I was going to do to make sense of what I was trying to achieve in order to define my research question. I still had big gaps in my understanding of what had occurred and what had happened to the rest of my colleagues. I had to know. And Sherlock was back in the building.

Unlike when writing a book of fiction, every fact within an academic thesis must be referenced or already in the public domain. There is no room for creative language or prose. This work is a structured publication that spells everything out, from the intent of the study, the methodology, the literature review, the evidence, then finally to the conclusion and recommendations for the future. This last sentence is a serious oversimplification on my part — trust me. I now know that understanding the expected framework of a thesis at PhD level is very different to undertaking a thesis at Master's level. I was guided by Jeanne Madison through the application to the Ethics Committee. Under her supervision, I made contact with the other nurses and gathered their written consent to participate in the research. Once all the consents were in hand, I started asking myself, in terms of definition of the research question, what it was that I wanted to prove. The requirement for any research degree is that it must add to that which is already known in the scientific community. I will admit, study at this level is onerous and even though I had researched and written a thesis before, I struggled to decide upon the how of it — how the interviews would be structured and what I hoped to garner from the nurses' stories. I was lost, so I mapped out what I already knew, and the way forward became obvious. My research questions became absolutely clear to me; we were a group of nurses who had been erroneously labelled as whistleblower nurses. We were all aware that we were publicly displayed with that label. My questions focussed not on nurses advocating for patients, but on nurses themselves and what, if any price, had they paid for truth-telling by unauthorised disclosure to the media.

The title of my research was: An Australian whistleblowing experience in healthcare: A study of six women from the New South Wales public health system who were labelled by the media as whistleblower nurses.

I conducted an extensive literature review searching for how my experience and (hopefully) the experiences of my colleagues would add to what was already known. I confirmed there were no other studies on a group of whistleblower nurses on the planet — this was unique research and is recognised as such. These were big questions that only found answers six years later, when the data was collected, collated and the thesis was written.

There were times I hated myself for the questions I knew I had to ask my colleagues, but I had a plan.

Logic is my friend. As I have already said, I am a person who likes order and straight lines, I loathe disorder and disarray. After the necessary permissions were garnered from both the university and the participants, I was ready to begin. This was a strange time for me. I knew what I wanted to prove, but how the hell did I get there? How did I know what the responses of the participants would be? What if I couldn't do this? The nagging fear of failure began to move like a gossamer wisp through my brain. I was determined to ignore it.

One of the conditions of the conduct of this research by the Ethics Committee was that it was my responsibility to ensure my colleagues were aware that participation in sensitive research could be damaging. I was required to include a statement about seeking professional help should reactions to participation in this research occur. At no time did I imagine this warning was applicable to me. I figured this was a 'rubber stamp' kind of thing that exonerated the University should any of the participants experience distress from being involved in the interview process. I could not have been more wrong. Again, naive.

I defined my interview strategy while I continued to immerse myself in working as a midwife. I now knew where I was going. I just needed to ask the right questions at the interviews to collect the information I needed. God, it was so good to immerse myself in study again. Twelve years prior, Professor Victor Minichiello gave a qualitative research lecture to my Bachelor of Health Management class. Since that time, I had been forever fascinated by how other people viewed the world. I knew my research methodology would be qualitative as I wanted to capture the individual nurses' experiences through their eyes, without judgement or any sanitation of the words. I wanted to hear it from them, first-hand, to enable me to understand and learn exactly what had happened to them. This distraction was a godsend for me and for a while, it provided me with balance while I worked on the Antenatal Ward.

My father's edict to "do the right thing" has stayed with me my entire life. I believe in fair play; I am a strong patient advocate. But sometimes, I wish I just didn't give a bugger. I wish I could just go to work with blinkers on, pretend everything was rosy, then go home and not give work or patients a second thought while enjoying my salary after it hit my bank account every fortnight. Unfortunately, for me, it just doesn't work that way. I wish sometimes I could be like that, to just turn and walk away. But then, as the saying goes 'if wishes were horses, then beggars would ride'. Do the blinkered people struggle with their Switzerland stance or do they in fact, truly believe as a lot of people say, 'it's not my problem?' I will never know, because that is not the type of person I am. I am well and truly on the other side of the fence. I report near misses, poor practice and adverse outcomes. In my experience, a good number of managers probably wish I would go the hell away and stop highlighting events that are complex and difficult to solve. In other words, not addressing or escalating information is a means of keeping the status quo — the status quo for them that is.

The pressure on public hospitals to get people out of Emergency Departments by either discharging them, or finding them a bed in the hospital is overwhelming for hospital patient flow managers. Nowadays, men and women are housed in the same four bedded wards. Muslim women are terrified, and their families are offended, but so long as bums are not in beds in the Emergency Department for longer than four hours and a Breach Report to the Department of Health is avoided, then it would seem the end justifies the means. Not bloody likely.

The Antenatal Ward became a conveniently labelled Women's Health Ward. We used to joke and say, "If you have a vagina, you will get a bed on this come one, come all ward".

This was disrespectful, I know but it was also true. Every patient on the ward was assigned to a midwife as the person responsible for their care. While endorsed enrolled nurses worked on this ward, they were not held responsible for the care of the patient and any concerns or issues were reported to the midwife.

Working on this ward often reminded me of being a circus juggler as the scope of patients ranged from the aged and demented, to teenagers who were too old for the Paediatric Ward. Primarily, the domain of the ward was for antenatal patients, but when the Emergency Department was full, any bed would do to prevent the dreaded Breach Report as a result of bed block.

I was of the view that the 'open bookings' policy of this maternity unit was also attributable to the imposition of considerable hardships imposed upon patients and midwives alike. One such scenario was that the manager of the

Antenatal Ward was expected to accept patients who, in other better resourced facilities, would have been managed with greater empathy. Patients with early trimester pregnancies whose foetus(s) had died or who were pregnant with a foetus with abnormalities were given the option to have a termination of pregnancy. This procedure did not involve a dilation and curettage (D&C) of the uterus under general anaesthetic. The patient was admitted to the Antenatal Ward with other expectant mothers happily awaiting the birth of their child. A Carnage pessary was inserted into the vagina at regular intervals to initiate labour, which like any other labour, was painful and distressing. For these women, even more so, because they were not going to birth a healthy, live baby to take home. It was just so hard. We grieved with the women and their partners. The other true horror for these women was that the Antenatal Ward was the 'overflow' ward when the Postnatal Ward was full. The sound of crying babies for these women must have been nothing short of torture. Their grief was a miasma that enveloped us all.

16

The sound of a woman keening after the death of a child has a pitch and timbre that is unique and beyond macabre. It is a sound that makes my blood run cold. Its resonance was burned into my brain as a student midwife and has been resurrected, again and again, every time I cared for one of these poor women. As midwives, we all grieved for the loss that was to come and shared in the deluge of pain that would descend upon this family. This process was so very difficult. Night after night, coming to work, dreading that a Carnage patient would be on the ward and then knowing, I would be caring for her and potentially, eleven other patients until the end of my shift; by which time the woman could have delivered her baby. In truth, none of us relished looking after these women as being exposed regularly to extreme grief is soul destroying. The grief of losing a baby weighs heavy on a midwife's heart.

No care for the psyche of the midwives. No understanding of the cause and effect of grief upon the staff caring for these women and how that grief like a vapour is absorbed and retained. I recall one particular woman who had elected to undergo a Cervagem termination of pregnancy that today, still plagues me. The foetus's life was terminated because on ultrasound, a cleft lip and palate was identified. The father of the child had been born with the same condition. He had endured numerous operations and the obvious scarring was a thing of horror for him. As a child, he had been stared at and had been tormented and teased mercilessly by other children. He did not want a child with a cleft lip and palate, so the decision was made to terminate the otherwise perfectly formed foetus. I struggled with this. To me, the decision of the medical officer to agree to terminate this child's life was morally and ethically wrong. I grieved for that child for a very long time.

Repeated care of women with dead babies becomes a thing of exhaustion and horror. I recall two particular midwives who would get really irritable if they were allocated to care for a woman receiving Cervagem. This made the shift even harder, listening to their constant whinging and crankiness, which of course was an expression of how hard they found caring for these women.

It was a frequent occurrence for those of us midwives who were allocated to care for these grieving women and their partners (yes, that's right, not all midwives, regardless of their seniority, were allocated to the care of patients receiving Cervagem). The chosen few were spared the horror of delivering dead babies shift after shift. Those of us who did care for these women knew all too well how hard it was, both personally and professionally. I now know that those feelings that we were left with at the end of the shift are cumulative and destructive. We were never given the opportunity to debrief or to vent the profound sadness that is part of being involved in the death of a child. The shift finished and we were expected to drive home and sleep, only to come back the next night and do it all over again.

I understand grief and I understand that any baby, be it one day post conception or at full term, when lost, is a catastrophic moment in the life of the woman and her family. But I do not condone this hospital's horrific process involved after the birth of the deceased child — the practice of which might be nation-wide for all I know. Years ago, if a baby died, handprints and footprints were inked onto a card and given to the parents as a memory of the lost child. Often parents would have bronze casts made of the footprints to keep as a treasure. Today however, the concept of providing the parents with memories, for me, is a truly grisly practice. My next statements will invoke howls of protest from midwives around the world.

Again — my memoir — my reality.

Often the foetus is very small. If less than 12 weeks gestation, Polaroid photos are taken and an attempt is made to ink hand and footprints onto a card with the details of the date, time of birth and the name of the parents. If the photos are refused, they are stored in the patient file, in case years later (which has happened), the mother changes her mind and wants the photos. For women who deliver babies with abnormalities who choose not to see the child; it is not uncommon for them to manifest images of some terrible monster in their minds, when in fact this is so very often not the truth. Often a photograph of the child is enough to relinquish the monster and put the nightmares to rest. The storage of photographs of deceased babies will present an issue for the future, given that medical records in the public system are now all electronic. But that is another problem for another day.

If the foetus is from 18 weeks gestation, the practice was not only to weigh the baby, but to measure the head circumference and the length (for the birth card) but also to dress the baby in pretty baby clothing. Each mother was given a beautiful memorial baby quilt, made by some skilled quilter unknown. There were boxes of clothes donated by women who knitted and sewed endlessly, making baby clothes to fit a tiny doll, right through to sizes appropriate for a full-term infant. The babies were dressed and wrapped in rugs and given back to their parents to spend time with their child. I will never know if my loathing of this process came from my traumatic experience in the mortuary all those years ago when I was a student nurse. But I really struggled with this process.

I appreciate the importance of grieving parents spending time with their lost child. It is heartbreaking but so very necessary. What I found hard to come to terms with was the macabre process of dressing the child in handmade clothing. It always reminded me of those terrible turn of the century black and white funeral photos of families, dressed in their Sunday best with their deceased family member propped up on a chair. To me it felt disrespectful. The baby stayed with the parents until they were ready to relinquish the child to be taken to the mortuary. Often parents would request the child be brought back to them from the mortuary and the grieving started all over again.

I found it absolutely horrifying when parents kept the dead child in the room with them in a refrigerated cot, sometimes for days, while the inevitable biological process of decomposition began. The parents took the cold baby out of the cot for cuddles then returned the child to the cot for preservation. I can only imagine what the visitors of these women thought when they entered the room to see a metal box plugged into the wall. If the parents chose not to keep the baby in the room with them, often the baby was brought back from the mortuary to the room for the benefit of the patient's visitors. I never had the opportunity to speak to any of these people as to how they felt about having a dead baby in the room after they had arrived with flowers and fruit baskets to offer their condolences. I will never know. Perhaps my perceptions are the product of traumas past and my own personal fears and perceptions.

I like night duty and am well suited to it, as I sleep well during the day. Our night duty team was pretty stable and for the most part, we all got on well. The work was a constant tug-o-war of emotions that was physically and emotionally draining for us as midwives. The assortment of patients was eclectic and finding emotional balance and professional appropriateness was often extremely difficult. On any one shift in the allocation of my 12 patients, I potentially could be allocated the care of a woman receiving Cervagem and everything that goes with that scenario, while also being allocated the care of at least one woman receiving Prostin — another drug used to induce labour. In another room there could be a woman who was grieving for a dead child, while in the next room, a woman was bursting with excitement that today, she would give birth to her long-awaited healthy baby.

Christ, it was so hard to be empathetic or enthusiastic according to what room I was in. I always likened these days to wearing the face of the Phantom of the Opera — one glowing with happiness, one contorted with tragedy. This model of care wasn't fair to anyone — the patients or the staff. The patients soon got to know that the 'butterfly plaque' on the door of any of the single rooms meant there was a woman inside who had lost a baby. For the first time in my life, I felt the joy of being a midwife sucked out of me.

As a self-preservation strategy, I immersed myself into the research for my PhD. As with my previous two tertiary degrees, I studied externally because I needed to work full time. Self-discipline is paramount with external study as there are no classmates to study with and no lecturers on hand, it is just a hard slog. When I think back to those times, I equate my approach to the interviews like that of a blind woman who tap, tap, tapped with a long stick, searching, ever searching, for a path forward. I decided to break the inquiry into three parts, which meant three rounds of interviews. I had audio taped the interviews for my master's thesis, so that at least was familiar ground for me. What I had learned from that experience is to ask open ended questions that are specific. I also learned to keep control of the conversation, after all, every single word spoken had to be transcribed, typed and returned to the participant for sign off that what had been recorded was what was actually said. I learned that hard lesson when, during the research for my Masters, I had to type 25,000 words for an interview that was, for the most part, just chat between myself and the participant. Note to self. Focus and stay on track.

My colleagues and I had lived this experience, so I knew it was a hell of a story. My challenge, dear readers, is to share those experiences and my perceptions with you. I undertook an extensive review of the literature. I was amazed to learn that for whistleblowers, be they police officers, politicians, nurses or street sweepers, the trajectory and the outcome is always the same. I also studied how to undertake semi structured in-depth interviews with open-ended, probing questions. I wanted to capture the nurses' words, experiences, perceptions, individual recollections and stories. It wasn't until I completed this research that I realised how brave these nurses were, to have told their truths and to have entrusted that information to me.

All of the nurses in this study were seasoned clinicians, each with more than 30 years' experience under their belts. I thought I understood how challenging these interviews would be for the nurses. I didn't even consider there would be any degree of difficulty for me, as the researcher. I have never been more wrong in my life. I also completely underestimated how difficult it would be for them to resurrect painful memories at my hand. I am forever grateful to them for agreeing to be subjected to such scrutiny regarding their experiences.

From the outset I identified a potential stumbling block. I had previously worked with four of the nurses and I had been employed in a more senior position than them. As we had a pre-existing relationship, I feared these nurses may have felt obliged to participate in the study. I was also aware of the potential for 'modified truths' based on my previous supervisorial relationship with them and the resulting power differential. This fact was put on the table in recognition of my responsibility to ensure their choice to participate was of free will and not out of any sense of coercion. We talked about our pre-existing relationships and agreed that if they felt any sense of me pressuring them for answers they were not prepared to give, they were to call the interview to a halt. I needed to be very certain that our past would not be a factor that would affect the research and that the participants were comfortable with this proviso before the consent forms were signed.

I wanted to do everything I could to ensure the participants were as comfortable as possible. It was important to meet them at a venue of their choosing, on their 'turf' if you like, to ensure they could speak freely and confidentially. They also called the shots in terms of times of availability. It was agreed that the interviews could always be rescheduled if a situation arose for them that made the interview date and/or time unsuitable. As it turned out, all of the interviews, at the request of the nurses, were conducted inside their individual private residences. It was interesting to note that on the visits for the second and subsequent interviews, the familiarity of the setting seemed to impact positively on the free flow of dialogue.

In this research I was both a participant and the researcher to which the term Participant Observer is appointed. I discovered this role within sensitive research is challenging; not only from the point of view that I, with my researcher hat on, was repeatedly exposed to sensitive data which had the potential to be harmful to me, but also from the guilt I was assailed by when I asked probing questions and got heartbreaking answers.

I have learned that in this type of research it is vital that the two roles undertaken by the researcher/subject are portrayed as recognisably separate entities. This decision was made to ensure I was able to be clearly identified as a participant within the group that was being studied. This stance also allowed my truths to be heard by identification as the speaker. The second voice allowed my experiences as the researcher to become another identifiable layer within the study. The distinction between these two roles was difficult to achieve but imperative to this research, if I was to be able to recount my own experiences as the author and a participant within the study.

The first round of interviews:

The purpose of the first round of interview questions was to improve my knowledge about each of the nurses as people and their understanding of:

a. The importance of truth telling

b. How and why they became a nurse.

c. What it means to be a nurse.

d. What happened to cause them to speak out publicly?

e. If they had their time again would they make the same choices again, and why?

Factual Accuracy Disclaimer: *The following text includes factual information and research-based content. The author has made every reasonable effort to ensure the reliability of sources and the accuracy of content. Readers are encouraged to verify the facts independently and consult authoritative sources if needed. The full version of the PhD version can be found: https://rune.une.edu.au/web/retrieve/0c966102-bdf7-40d1-9af6-f619385ff0fd*

The participants:

Monique: Aged forty-nine this year. Divorced with three kids, all grown up. I've been a nurse for many years. I started nursing in 1975. I finished [registered nurse training] in '78. I've worked in a lot of hospitals in a major metropolitan Area Health Service and the private [system] ... I became a nurse because I wanted to help people. When my father died, I just wanted to give back to people what was taken from me — actually wanted to be a policeman. I had a lot of anger and I wanted to be a policeman because you have the gun and you have the power ... but I chose nursing. I was one of those difficult children. I was labelled. If my dad was alive, I would have shoved my [nursing] certificate up his nose because he always led me to believe that I would never amount to anything ... and I have ... I think I have achieved my goal, helping people, being a patient advocate and a staff advocate.

Meadhbh: I am fifty-five years old, divorced in recent times with two grown children. I can remember the day that I went for my interview to be a nurse. In those days it was expected that you wore hats and gloves and looked very proper in your suit ... and I didn't, I wore a summer dress, which was a mini skirt! I sat in a sitting room with other girls in their brown suits [chuckle] and their gloves and their hats and the sun was splitting the rocks. They were hot and bothered and said, 'You are wasting your time here; they are not going to give you your training here'. I walked into the room and the panel said, 'You are like a breath of sunshine'. I did of course get into St James [hospital] in Dublin. I did my finals in '71 then I did my maternity in the Maternity hospital and stayed on for five years. Then I went on to St James operating theatres and I moved out to Australia eleven years ago.

Violet: I am soon to be thirty-nine, divorced with one child who is nearly eleven. Nursing to me wasn't just a job; it was really a passion for me. I absolutely loved it ... it was my contribution to the world. I did my Bachelor of Applied Science (Nursing) at university ... I went back [to university] for two years part time to do the degree ... then I did the coronary care course. I immediately after coming out of uni got a job at my local hospital on the new nurses' program. I did my last three months in Intensive/Coronary Care and of course I liked it and never looked back. I finished my Intensive and Coronary Care course and became a clinical nurse specialist. I just liked being on the floor [working as a clinician]. I also loved education.

Yanaha: I am 49 years old. I have three daughters and a husband. I am a nurse and I have been a nurse since I was sixteen years old. Nursing is an integral part of me, of who I am. I started nursing at sixteen, as a cadet nurse. I applied to do my training at a major Sydney referral hospital during 1974 and I was accepted. I didn't like nursing at all. In fact, I hated it. I was eighteen by then and I thought Nuh! I've made a mistake; this isn't what I should be doing. Then about half way through second year, when I was just about to throw it in, I did my first theatre term. I just remember walking in there, getting changed into scrubs and feeling like I had come home!

Simone: I am thirty-seven years old and was born in Sydney Australia. I am the eldest of three children. I have been married for thirteen years. I have been with my husband for twenty years. We have one daughter – she's seven. All of my adult life I have been nursing. I trained at a Sydney hospital in the 80's. I am a Buddhist. I am a very loyal person and I have quite high morals and a protective nature. I can't stand injustice or intolerance or things like that. I can be quite outspoken in defence of people, not usually for my own defence, but for the defence of people who I feel need my defending. I am an enrolled nurse...

Kathrine: I am aged fifty something, happily married for more than two decades with two remarkable children. I am a nurse dinosaur. At seventeen, in 1975, I started my nursing training at a rural facility through the hospital training system. I completed my general training in 1978, and midwifery training in 1979 and throughout my career, from clinician to senior manager I have been greatly influenced by my father's edict 'do it right the first time girl or don't do it at all!' As an Australian—a race known for 'doing the right thing', did those words set me on an impossible course to constantly seek truth and social justice not only in my own practice but also in the practice of others? Perhaps.

Narissa: (A non-participant in this study, – but a highly influential person). Information pertaining to Narissa is included in this research as she deliberately sought out each of the nurses to gain their stories which she released to the media without the knowledge or consent of the nurses. She was invited to participate in this research, however declined the offer, stating she had been traumatised by the events and had been advised by her doctor that participation in this study was not in her best interests.

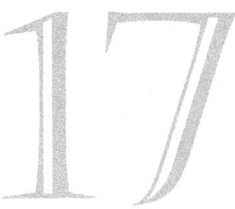

Professional transparent practice is an important tenet of nursing care. The nurses all shared their views on the value of the truth.

Question: How important is truth telling to you?

Monique: That is why I became a nurse. I am not going to hide things under the carpet. We do make mistakes, but we can learn from those mistakes as well.

Meadhbh: I am going to be very honest. I think that is the one thing that has got me through and made me hold my head up high is that I have always told the truth and have been found in the reports to have told the truth.

Violet: I just did what I needed to do to assist in keeping it going and to tell the truth.

Yanaha: They asked me questions and I told them the truth.

Simone: I told the truth 100%. I never deviated from my story;

I never changed my story. ICAC looked into everything I said ... they couldn't say anything but that I told the truth, because I did.

Kathrine: I did my job. I reported the truth as it had been reported to me.

Discussion: Truth telling is subjective, for individual reality equates to that person's perceived version of truth. Truth telling also has a dark side. It is commonly claimed that to unburden oneself by telling the truth is cathartic and healing. The literature also states the act of expressing life experiences to others can be a 'therapeutic benefit' when participating in sensitive research. My findings in no way support this supposition. However honourable, the decision to speak out publicly should never be undertaken lightly. The usual consequence for public declarations of poor patient care or adverse outcomes is public vilification, ostracism and marginalisation for the nurse. Truth telling comes at a high price.

Question: What did nursing mean to you prior to the whistleblowing event?

Monique: I became a nurse ... I wanted to help people.

Yanaha: I liked the idea of only having to look after one patient at one time and being able to actually focus your attention as part of the team on that patient's care — and giving that patient the best care possible.

Meadhbh: I loved the work so much I would do it without being paid.

Violet: Even though my love was Coronary Care, I loved the intensity of Intensive Care – with ventilators and multi-organ failure. I loved them both and I thought it was the best possible world I could get having both.

Simone: Absolute number one [priority] before a pan, before a pill, before a PhD ... the number one job of a nurse is patient advocacy. Your patient is your child.

Kathrine: By nature, I am a nurturer, so nursing was a profession that appealed to me. Nursing to me is caring for others the way you would want your own family cared for. Nursing is also about honour, integrity and truth.

We all shared the common view that caring is an important tenet for the profession of nursing and is inextricably linked to being a good nurse. As teenagers, we all entered the profession based on the value we attached to the role of the nurse and their contribution to society.

Question: Why did you become a nurse?

Monique: I am a patient and staff advocate who is a worker who takes pride in her work. It [honesty] is really, really important for the healing process and the grieving process, that families can see that we [nurses] did everything possible. I became a nurse 'cause I never had that with my father when he died.

Meadhbh: I can remember from the early days training at St James in Dublin which was the school of hard knocks on the floor, saying that I loved the work so much I would do it without being paid ... and that is something that stayed with me until I came and worked in NSW.

Violet: Nursing to me wasn't just a job. It was really a passion for me. I absolutely loved it. It was passion ... it was my contribution to the world.

Yanaha: During my general training ... I didn't like nursing at all. In fact I hated it. I didn't like the Army style regimentation that we were subjected to. Then about half way through second year, when I was just about to throw it in, I did my first theatre term. This was where I belonged. I am comfortable and I like this.

Simone: I am an enrolled nurse. I was hospital trained ... I did ten years of Oncology and Palliative Care [nursing] at a Sydney hospital. I had a very unique role. It was a very small unit ... I was very well educated. I used to give all of my own arterial chemotherapy, did all of my own cannulations, gave all my own oral and IM [intramuscular] medications ... everything ... except Schedule 8 drugs.

Kathrine: I have always believed nursing to be a very honourable profession; however, the expectation of subservience has for me been a lifelong challenge. Using science to help patients and their relatives has always appealed to me. I am a hypervigilant person who takes the responsibility of patient advocacy and patient safety very seriously. Nursing to me was never just a job. Until being labelled and punished as a whistleblower, it was the focus of my life.

It was clear all of the nurses were all passionate about their jobs which seemed to be a natural course for them and their way of life. Caring and advocacy for patients was a common finding.

Question: What were the circumstances that led to raising issues of concern with your employer?

Monique: In Intensive Care, a patient had undergone an aorto-femoral bypass that had gone wrong. She was intubated, ventilated and sedated but she wasn't dying. This particular doctor...who I had previously held suspicions about, went to the bed area and pulled the curtain around the woman. I was suspicious about what he was doin' at the head of the bed. I heard an alarm and I thought to myself 'Shit! What's going on?' I got up and saw bradycardia [slow heart rate on the monitor]. I went to resuscitate the patient when the doctor walks out and says, 'Don't worry' [dusting his hands together]. He walked away and didn't resuscitate this patient and I am going 'What just happened?

What the fuck just happened?' I was left to prepare the body. It wasn't until I started getting rid of things around the bed area ... I found the empty syringe ... on a syringe pump. It was then that it dawned on me! He must have caused her bradycardia by bolusing [deliberately administering a bolus dose] to the patient. That's why he walked away, because he knew I knew what he had done. We had another 'tubed' patient [patient waiting for a ventilator bed]. We had to either find another nurse or get rid of a patient! It was a simple as that!

Meadhbh: During my first year of employment, we had this patient for elective surgery on an abdominal aortic aneurysm. I was in charge that morning and I said to the surgeon that one of the grafts was not available on site and that I would need to get one from St. Elsewhere. He said no he didn't need it, so we opened [the patient] and cross-clamped the aorta. That was when the surgeon said that he needed the particular graft that we didn't have. We ended up finding one and ordered a taxi to get there to pick it up. By the time the graft came and we put it in and unclamped the aorta, it was two hours. The time allowed for cross clamping is one hour. It took the patient about two months to die ... it was the most appalling death.

There was the scenario of the anaesthetic registrar who was on the phone discussing a fourteen-year-old boy with a history of a relative who, as a consequence of malignant hyperthermia, had died on the operating table ... this [discussion about the patient] was happening at our front door and I thought that this should not be happening. When the anaesthetic registrar came off the phone ... she got really annoyed with me ... The consultant anaesthetist was called in. The surgeon came and it was agreed that they would try to get the child to St Elsewhere. The surgeon rang, got a bed for surgery the next day and that was fine, so everybody was happy. The next thing I knew which was a couple of days later when a Human Resources person came down to theatre and said to me that a complaint had been lodged about me and it was from the anaesthetic registrar. I got this three-page document of allegations against me and they stood me down.

Violet: A patient came to Intensive Care from Delivery Suite. We were told she was an asthmatic in respiratory distress and that she was thirty-six weeks [pregnant]. Eventually the obstetric registrar came in. He wouldn't do the Caesar [caesarean section] because there was too much of a risk as the patient was too unstable. I remember the anaesthetic registrar yelling at him and me begging him, but he just wouldn't do it. So the anaesthetic registrar said, 'Well we are going to have to ship her out then'. I left the obstetric registrar to phone Care Flight. Time went past and I said to the anaesthetic registrar, 'They [Care Flight] aren't here yet. So off I went to ring them. The [Care Flight doctor's] response was, 'Oh that ... No that doctor cancelled that, he said you and the other doctor were over reacting and that she was fine.' I said, 'Oh my God, oh my God, [voice pleading] please just listen to me.' I heard him yell, 'Gear up! Gear up! We're going! ... The patient was on the brink of death and so was the baby. The mother survived and the baby was born with zero Apgars [Numerical score indicating neonatal wellbeing at birth, 5 minutes and 10 minutes of age]. The mother survived with a baby that has profound cerebral palsy.

Yanaha: One weekend, one of the surgeons turned up obviously affected by alcohol. An RN who was working with me said, 'Dr X just pulled up and I went over to have a smoke with him and he's pissed! He was coming to do an appendix on a child'. The RN went and said [to Dr X], 'Mate you're pissed!' and he said, 'No I just had a glass of wine at lunch, but I am not pissed. I'm fine. I'm fine to operate'. We got called back at about 10 o'clock at night for a child with a torsion of a testicle. The Emergency Department nurse said to me, 'Listen, I just watched him [Dr X] get out of his car and he is staggering drunk!' I said, 'Oh my God, he was three sheets to the wind at lunch time, imagine what he is going to be like at eleven o'clock at night!' The RN and I went round to the Emergency Department to find the anaesthetist, Doctor X and parents of the child. The RN and I said to the surgeon, 'Now look! You can't even stand up straight. Why don't you do this case tomorrow morning? Why don't you put it on the end of your list tomorrow?' The anaesthetist said the kid hadn't fasted long enough and the surgeon said 'Alright, we'll do it tomorrow.'

Meadhbh and I put together a conference called 'Learning to Love the Law'. There were a couple of doctors, a couple of nurses and the General Manager on the panel. I gave them all names and different roles [from the roles they normally undertook]. I sort of gave them the hierarchy of the chess set, i.e. the surgeon was Dr King, the anaesthetist was Dr Queen, the resident was Dr Knight and the role I assigned to the General Manager was that of the pawn. I called her Virginia Pawn (probably interpreted as Virginia Porn). I posed a scenario and I asked her, 'Well what are you going to do Virginia?' She was staring at the audience; I am not even sure if she was listening to me. I said, 'Hallo ... hallo ... wakey, wakey are you with us Virginia ... you know Sister Pawn?' We never intended to make her look foolish. However, the feedback at the end of the day was that the audience thought that we made a fool of her and that she would be out to get us. I have no proof of this but...

Simone: I was always a bit fan of the MET [Medical Emergency Team] system. As soon as a patient's blood pressure reaches a certain point, you can call this MET and they will act before the patient is [mortally] compromised. I had a patient with terrible sleep apnoea. He was very obese ... We rang the doctor ... maybe three times. I said to him on the last occasion, 'I am going to call a MET... He said, 'Call a MET all you want cause I am the only doctor in the hospital and I ain't comin'! I am busy!' I tried everything ... felt so helpless, so I said, 'Why not try the Laerdal bag over his face and just pretend?'... He breathed in ... after about a minute ... he calmed down and went to sleep. A couple of days later [sigh] at the disciplinary interview I was advised I had acted outside of my scope of practice.

I had this lady who had come into hospital dreadfully unwell ... I called a MET... The doctor came up from ICU and came charging into the room... then he goes [away]. I ring again and the MET came back up. The doctor asked, 'What are you calling me again for?' 'Because she has gotten worse'. So he goes up to the patient ... and said [in a very loud voice], 'You don't want to live, do you? You don't want us to put a tube down your throat, do you? You don't want us to be pumping on your chest and doing all that do you'? She says, 'Bloody oath I do'! He tried to coerce her to document herself as not for resuscitation. I said to him, 'What are you doing'? He said, 'I don't have a bed. What do you want me to do nurse? Pull one out of my arse'? I had called a MET three times by this stage and he said, 'Don't call me again'!

I stood watching her deteriorate and she said, 'Please Simone ... don't let me die ... don't let me die'. I said, [Simone burst into tears, sobbing now] 'I promise I won't'. And then I thought I can't do this anymore! I can't do it! I grabbed the bed, got to the lift and pushed through the doors of ICU ... I saw this nurse with long hair [Violet]. Later I got a phone call from this nurse. 'Oh, are the nurse that brought Mrs So and So down to ICU?' I said, 'Yeah'. She said, 'Oh I am really sorry, but she's dead'. And I said, 'No shit'!

Kathrine: I was working as an After-Hours Senior Nurse Manager at a New South Wales tertiary referral hospital. Monique [participant in this study] in her capacity as a highly experienced intensive care nurse reported to me that a senior Intensive Care Unit doctor had deliberately terminated the life of an elderly female postoperative patient by injecting her with the contents of a full syringe of narcotics. The rationale for this action was to 'free up' an otherwise unavailable ventilator bed for a young male who had undergone emergency surgery. In my role as the After- Hours Senior Nurse Manager, I was obliged to report this sentinel event. This tragedy was made even more profound when the young male died on the operating table.

All of the nurses advocated for their patients to protect them from harm. To do so is the expected role of a professional nurse—innate behaviour. We now know that advocacy is a huge risk. If a patient's condition changes or looks like they might come to harm, we all went out on a limb to protect them. Little did we know there is no safety net for us when advocating for patients.

Question: Why did you speak out?

Simone: I just thought I was being a patient advocate, identifying to colleagues that the practices that were going on were not in the best interest of the patient.

Yanaha: This is a problem, patients are coming to harm, somebody needs to do something and if not me then who? Because no one else was doing anything.

Meadhbh: It was quite clear that the case was going to go ahead had I not intervened ... and I mean maybe the kid would have been alright ... and maybe he wouldn't, and we are not there to take those kinds of risks.

Violet: When you know that sort of stuff you have obligation ... not just an obligation, but morally you do the right thing.

Monique: For the same reason I became a nurse ... I wanted to help people.

Kathrine: Nursing was my life. I am warrior born so it is in my nature to defend and protect. For me I can never just turn my back and walk away.

All public hospitals are required to report information to NSW Health about extreme adverse outcomes such as suicide of an inpatient, the wrong blood being transfused and a myriad of other serious events that may or may not have been attributed to human error, equipment failure or an unavoidable but foreseeable possibility. There is a plethora of literature that confirms an epidemic of under-reported, preventable injuries to patients. In my experience the reasons for keeping a lid on adverse outcomes is primarily to ensure the public retains faith in its hospitals and services. However, it is imperative to keep silent if senior managers are to avoid the attention of New South Wales Health. Non-disclosure of errors is a highly effective way of deflecting insurance claims, preventing adverse career trajectory and deceiving the public that it serves. It is far more acceptable for senior managers to lay blame at the feet of an individual or a group of individuals than to take responsibility for known problems and adverse outcomes.

18

I felt as though there were two Kathrines – Kathrine the midwife, and Kathrine the PhD student. When I was Kathrine the midwife I was working four ten-hour shifts a week. I was regularly in charge of my shift and was often deployed to areas such as the Delivery Suite if they were short-handed, which was a joy to me as I loved working in Delivery. When I was Kathrine the PhD student, my time was spent slavishly transcribing the words of my colleagues into hard copy.

The fourth question of the first round of interviews confirmed for me that we are all patient advocates who accept the welfare of our patients as an absolute personal responsibility.

God, qualitative research is exciting!

Question: If you had the opportunity to go back to a time prior to the events that happened to you, would you make the same choices?

Monique: Bloody oath I would. That is why I became a nurse. I am not going to hide things under the carpet. We do make mistakes, but we can learn from those mistakes as well. I would do it again. I wouldn't not say anything because I would not let that bastard [the ICU doctor] get away with that. I have to live with my conscience. On my deathbed, I can say to myself, 'Well Monique you tried. At least you tried. You didn't pretend it didn't happen.' I am a worker ... I won't put those blinkers on. I won't do it. I may as well get out of nursing.

Meadhbh: Well, that is a question that I ask myself over and over because ... what happened had a huge impact upon my life. So much has changed in my life. The bottom line is I never saw myself as a whistleblower. I was somebody who was doing what I believed to be the right thing. I know that some people used this opportunity to damage me and I think ... in all ... I don't think they expected the outcome to be as serious [as it turned out to be]. I don't believe they wanted me to be this destroyed, but I know that they wanted to shut me up. In answer to this question and this is the interesting thing, this is a terrible thing that has happened. But I couldn't not do it, because it is how I ... it's how I look after my patients ... I say no, this is wrong. It is also the personality I have too in that I am not afraid to speak up.

Violet: Was it worth it – no, because nothing really changed. But would I do it again? Yes. When you know that sort of stuff you have not just an obligation, but a moral obligation ... morally you must do the right thing. You want to do the right thing. So I would do it again, but I would just be more … if I had the knowledge I have now, I would not be so naive and I would know to write down everything … to have collected more information like Narissa did … yeah that is the only thing I would do differently.

Yanaha: Well, it wasn't a choice really. It wasn't something that I made a conscious choice about. Patients were coming to harm, somebody needed to do something and if not me, then who? Because no-one else was doing anything. That's what I don't agree with. I can't stand people who just turn a blind eye. I can't stand to do it myself … I can't do it. It is not a choice; it is just something that you feel is right. I was just being a nurse as far as I was concerned … I was just doing my job! So I would have to say I would do the same thing because it is not a choice.

Simone: Every time! Every single time! You could ask me that in ten years or in twenty years or in one hundred years and it is never going to change! But I hate to say this, it has changed me. I have seen things since that I haven't reported. If that had happened before, I would have reported it. But this has taught me you can't change everyone's practice and that if you practise the same way consistently every time, often the people around you will change their practice because they realise that they can do it better.

Kathrine: I did my job to the best of my ability and it was to my absolute detriment. I exposed the truth about the patient who was allegedly 'terminated' by an ICU doctor; a truth that would otherwise not have come to light. Would I make the same choices again? For the most part I would say yes, however we struggle to make ends meet because I no longer earn the type of income I used to earn. Also, when the blackness and the fear return and consume me, I struggle with it. But after everything that has come to pass, I feel no guilt. I did my job as a nurse and I sleep at night. I know I told the truth and for what it is worth in the face of a ruined career and an acquired life-long acute anxiety disorder, if a patient came to harm and the local management didn't step up, would I speak out again? God help me, yes.

After speaking with each of the nurses, during this first round of interviews, one theme became patently clear; we didn't regard ourselves as whistleblowers. None of us actually spoke out publicly until after the various recounts of adverse clinical outcomes were released by Narissa. As professional nurses, we each spoke out because of expected professional conduct, good faith, beneficence, moral responsibility and the Australian cultural ethic "to do the right thing". Maternalism was an obvious motivating factor for Simone. It became clear that doing the right thing was important to each of us, as we all had unwavering faith in the reporting and investigation process of our employing facilities and the responsibility of senior managers to act upon that advice for the betterment of patient care. It seems our beliefs in the system were little more than naivety.

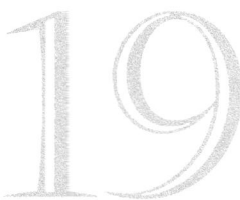

19

Finally, the first round of interviews were complete and the onerous task of converting taped conversation into text seemed to take an eternity. Now it was time for me to absorb the information from the first round of interviews and focus on building the questions for the second round while continuing to work as a full-time night duty practicing midwife.

It was hard to stay focussed and energised when the level of deskill for this workforce was well known and never addressed. Inequity was an issue for clinicians on the Antenatal Ward, not only in terms of patient allocation but also with deployment. There were only two of us on night duty that were regularly deployed to Delivery Suite. The other midwives claimed they were out of practice as they hadn't delivered a baby for more than 20 years. Only one other midwife was rotated to Delivery Suite to up-skill. So much for the definition of a midwife ... an accountable professional who works in partnership with women to give the necessary support, care and advice during pregnancy, labour and the post-partum period, to conduct birth on the midwife's own responsibility and to provide care for the newborn and the infant.

I will never understand why these midwives were not supervised and mentored to become more skilled. Better still, why did they not step up in recognition of needing to increase their own skill set? These midwives still put their hands out at the end of each fortnight and took the wages associated with possessing a midwifery qualification and the necessary skills required to be registered to practice as a midwife. The skills issue was an ongoing source of animosity between midwives. The management used a band-aid strategy when a voluntary rotation to Delivery Suite was offered to all midwives. Let me say there was no stampede to take up this opportunity. The management of this service did not realise the quantum gap involved in reducing workforce stagnation to empowerment with updated skills. The organisation did nothing to create a transition program for the midwives to give them an opportunity to work in a supported environment and gain the skills that are required to work across the midwifery continuum. However, there was no address of this issue—another addition to the too hard basket.

I struggled with being broken but I functioned as a professional midwife bolstered by decades of experience. A 30-something year old midwife who was known by the management to have less than stellar clinical skills embroiled me in a situation that I will always believe was caused by her lack of skills.

A young woman was admitted to the ward for Prostin induced labour. The attending midwife had been proven to be less than competent with undertaking of vaginal assessments in the past. Information gained from the vaginal exam must be accurate —the dilation of the cervix, the station (how high or low the baby is in the vaginal canal) and the position the baby was in, which is discerned by palpation of the fontanelles (the soft spots on newborn babies' heads).

There was a protocol for the administration of Prostin by an accredited midwife. If, on vaginal examination, any of the parameters were outside of protocol range, a medical officer was called and the decision was made whether or not to induce labour.

The midwife's documented findings of the vaginal examination were within the range of the protocol. She proceeded and administered the Prostin.

As a routine, midwives were allocated a group of patients at the beginning of our working week and we kept those patients for continuity of patient care. However, this night, the midwife who had been allocated to the group of patients that this young woman was in was deployed to the Postnatal Ward for the shift which meant the allocation had to be reshuffled. I ended up with the young woman who had received the Prostin in my allocation.

The patient was soon in established labour and was coping well. Her partner was with her and he was very supportive. A couple of hours later it was clear to me that she was ready to go to Delivery Suite as she was needing more pain relief than was permitted to be administered on the ward. I packed up her things and rang the Delivery Suite to advise I was transferring the patient to them, only to be advised, sorry there is no room. I informed the couple and assured them the Delivery Suite were aware of the advanced stage of her labour.

Not long afterwards, the partner came looking for me and informed me his girlfriend was sitting on the toilet. His face was pinched with anxiety when he said, "There's something hanging out, I think it's the umbilical cord."

I dropped everything and ran. He was right. The umbilical cord was visible, hanging out of the vagina. I got the woman back to bed, positioned her on all fours — head down — bum up, hit the emergency button and performed a vaginal examination. There was nothing in the pelvis! That is how the cord had prolapsed. The Delivery Suite was notified, and the Registrar instructed the person on the phone to bring the patient to the Delivery Suite.

I felt the patient needed to go to operating theatres NOW, for an emergency caesarean section. The registrar, who clearly had no faith in my ability to know a cord prolapse when I encountered one, insisted the patient be transferred to Delivery

Suite. I couldn't believe it! This went against everything I had ever been trained to do. The patient was transferred on the bed, still head down, bum up with me perched on the bed with my fingers in her vagina pushing the presenting part off the pulsating cord.

When we got to Delivery Suite and the cord was visible, the decision was made to go to theatres STAT for an emergency caesarean section. When the woman was transferred to theatres, she was manoeuvred from the ward bed to the operating table. My fingers were still pressed hard up against the presenting part to allow the blood to keep pulsating to this foetus. I was aware of the Neonatal team in the corner, setting up to receive the baby. The woman was anaesthetised and the drape that created the sterile field went over my head. I prayed the scalpel didn't slice through my fingers as claustrophobia engulfed me. I have never been good with enclosed spaces so I closed my eyes and just focused on breathing.

"I must not fear.

Fear is the mind-killer.

Fear is the little-death that brings total obliteration.

I will face my fear.

I will permit it to pass over me and through me.

And when it has gone past, I will turn the inner eye to see its path.

Where the fear has gone there will be nothing.

Only I will remain."

Once the incision was made and the baby was lifted out of the uterus. I came out from under the drape, sweating, panicked and numb. I looked at the white floppy, compromised body of this otherwise perfectly healthy baby and for a while, I just ceased to be.

I was aware the baby had been removed from the operating room on the resuscitation trolley. All eyes were on me. I pulled off my gloves and walked out of the theatre into the corridor. I encountered the partner who was standing alone in the corridor. He was frantic and crying. I had blood on my scrubs and my feet just didn't want to function. He grabbed my hand, "How is she? How is she? Is everything alright? How is the baby?"

The paralysis of brokenness descended upon me. I could barely speak. The most I could manage was, "Your partner has had an emergency caesarean section. The baby is very unwell. I am so terribly sorry."

I started to cry and the tears didn't stop. I went back to the ward, still dressed in my blood-soaked scrubs and someone paged the After-Hours Manager. We sat and talked for a long time. I couldn't continue on with the shift. She didn't want me to drive home as I was in no condition to be behind the wheel of a car. All I wanted to do was to vomit. I remember someone gave me a green plastic basin in case I had to vomit on the drive home. I had to get out of there.

When I got home, nothing seemed comforting or familiar. I didn't sleep. The next morning, the house had once again become a vacuum and I ran outside to be able to breathe. The traumas of the past and the fact that I had cared for a woman whose baby had come to terrible harm through no fault of my own, I knew was a professional noose around my neck and the drop platform was about to give way underneath me. The demons were back.

My husband was beyond terrified that this event was the one that would push me over the edge and I would take my own life. He was like a second skin and didn't leave my side. I went back to my GP. I don't remember anything else, except he said I was not to return to work for the next foreseeable future. I guess my husband faxed the GP's information to someone, because I received a call from the Acting Senior Nurse Manager of the Division. She was kind and empathetic and recommended I stay home and seek help.

I had to ask. I had to know the outcome for the baby. She paused for a very long time. I waited and held my breath, waiting for her answer. The baby had died of in-utero asphyxiation as a result of the cord prolapse.

I don't remember a lot of the next few weeks. I don't know when my brain actually started to function again. Suddenly I recalled the vaginal examination I had performed on the woman when the cord prolapse was first discovered. There was no head in the pelvis! This meant when the midwife examined the woman, her estimations were inaccurate. The presenting part would have been far too high to consider administering Prostin, due to the risk of cord prolapse. I knew the cord prolapse was not of my doing, but it didn't take the guilt of a dead baby away.

I still grieve for this woman and the loss of her precious child, but the professional guilt I felt, was put to rest. The Nursing Unit Manager of the Antenatal ward, not once, ever picked up the phone to inquire how I was coping. Once we had been friends and colleagues.

Several weeks later the Acting Senior Nurse Manager of the Division offered me a job managing accreditation for the service—a strategy to get me back to work. She realised it was still too early for me to consider returning to the clinical environment. I worked in this role for a few months, and it was helpful to be back working with people I knew, albeit in a different capacity. Finally, I decided it was time to go back to working on the Antenatal Ward as a midwife.

After a few weeks, I was summoned to the office of the Delivery Suite Manager for a meeting with her and the newly appointed Area Senior Nurse Manager. It seems I was to be held accountable for the management of the cord prolapse, despite the fact that I didn't administer the Prostin, and that I didn't give the order to transfer the patient to the Delivery Suite. A midwife does not have the delegated authority to arrange for a surgical procedure, which is the sole responsibility of the medical officer. Regardless, I was scapegoated as the protocol for management of a cord prolapse by taking the patient straight to theatre was not followed. There was no discussion regarding the administration of the Prostin. My punishment was to be seconded to work day shift in Delivery Suite to be supervised and mentored, with an evaluation of my clinical abilities. After the second day, I was allocated patients of my own, unsupervised. At the end of the first week the Nursing Unit Manager of the Delivery Suite asked, "Kath, what the hell are you doing here?"

To this day, I wish someone had informed this couple that their baby had died because the midwife got it wrong and that the Prostin should never have been administered; that the presenting part was too high and the risk of cord prolapse was too great. The matter would never have gotten to court and the parents would have known the truth. But someone had to be held accountable. If someone was not to blame, the organisation would be forced to investigate the finer details of the event and report to NSW Health. The organisation would be held accountable for allowing a midwife with known competency issues to administer Prostin.

The Nursing Unit Manager of the ward would have been held liable for inadequate supervision and mentorship of this midwife and the Division, had the incident been reported to New South Wales Health, would have been under fire for poor management of clinical skills and blinkered leadership.

The Antenatal Ward frequently had patients admitted who were incarcerated at the local prison. There were two levels of prisoners — those from the minimum-security area and those from the place for more extreme offenders. The latter would be handcuffed to the bed, despite a guard being posted. I always looped the nurse call bell around the bed rail within easy reach of the patient. A number of these guards were power hungry masochists. I was always sure to make very regular rounds of these women, who I knew were prone to mistreatment or taunting by the guards.

I will never forget one woman, handcuffed to the bed with one male and one female guard at her bedside. I made my rounds to ensure the patient was comfortable. The first thing I noticed was that all the lights were blazing. The second thing I noticed was that the nurse call bell was nowhere to be seen. I went over and began to reattach the bell to the bedrail, when the female guard grabbed my hand and said, "Don't do that, she'll ring the bell all night long. I'll call you if she needs anything." I smiled at the patient who was clearly very upset as I finished reattaching the nurse call bell. I asked the patient if she needed anything. She asked me for a drink of water. That was when I noticed her water jug had been moved out of arms reach. I took the jug, filled it with iced water and brought it back to the patient with a clean tumbler. I filled the glass with water which she gulped down like someone who had been left exposed in the desert. I poured her another which she also drank. She then settled back down on the bed, and I addressed the officers as I turned out the glaring overhead lights. "This patient may be incarcerated, but while she is a patient on this ward, I am in charge. The lights are to remain off, the water jug is to be within hands reach and the nurse call bell is to be available to the patient at all times."

The smart mouthed female guard said, "Well you'll be bloody sorry. She'll ring the bell all night long."

My response was, "This patient is entitled to the same civil liberties as any other citizen in this country. I'll check in regularly."

I then spoke to the patient, "If you need anything, just press the call bell and I will be the one to respond."

I didn't hear from her for the rest of the night. I called the jail and spoke to the person in-charge and complained about the treatment these two guards had meted out against this defenceless woman. I put in an incident report which apparently did not warrant a reply.

20

There are some patients who are never forgotten. In 2006, a woman was admitted to the Antenatal Ward because of a placental complication. She had been an inpatient for a long period of time. I always felt for her and her husband and their other children as they were country people who lived a long way from the hospital. When patients are in hospital for an extended period of time, the staff get to know them and their family. This woman was lovely. I recall she was so tiny with this little pregnant bump. She was less than 50kgs at 37 weeks gestation. After an event on the day shift, it was decided that the patient would be delivered by caesarean section. The theatre nurses alerted at least two medical staff of their concerns for this patient. These concerns were dismissed, and the patient was delivered of a little girl.

After the patient returned to the ward, the midwives became concerned that her blood pressure was very low. A junior resident responded to the call for assistance and prescribed intravenous fluids. The resident was then paged several times. On arrival, the resident, without consultation with a more senior medical officer, continued to order more intravenous fluids. Some hours later during the afternoon shift, a Patient Controlled Analgesia (PCA) pump with a morphine loaded syringe was commenced.

    The night shift had taken handover when the emergency buzzer blared like a Klaxon from the Postnatal Ward. That particular night, fortunately, there were three midwives rostered to the Antenatal Ward. All three of us responded to the call. The flashing light blinked red outside a single room at the end of the corridor. I was the second respondent and I will never forget the look on the midwife's face who was performing CPR on a woman who was clearly dead. The patient was so pale, she looked as though she had exsanguinated (died from a lack of blood). I pulled back the sheet expecting to see a massive postpartum haemorrhage — nothing but a tiny clot at the introitus of the vagina. The midwife who was performing CPR and whom I knew well and had a great deal of respect for, was wide eyed, disbelief painted on her face. Her actions were robotic, drawn from years of annual CPR training. She kept doing cardiac compressions while I bagged oxygen into the patient's lungs. The Medical Emergency Team (MET) arrived. Everyone was shocked. This was a Postnatal Ward — a happy place with women and their new babies, a dead woman was most unexpected. It was also a sentinel event.

The resuscitation continued until the medical Team Leader declared the patient dead and the time of death was recorded. Later, the midwife who was performing CPR told me the midwife who was actually allocated to the patient had approached her soon after the commencement of the shift and whispered, "You need to come. I think Patient X is dead."

The midwife she informed immediately went to the patient's room and started CPR. The allocated midwife turned and walked away, then disappeared into the ether.

The final investigation found that the patient had been unobserved for two hours prior to death, excessive soft tissue blood loss at the time of caesarean section and morphine toxicity as the potential causes of death. I, along with others involved that night, was required to attend the Coroner's Court for the hearing. I will never forget the look of absolute anguish on the patient's husband's face. He was a farmer with a dead wife and other small children, plus a new baby to rear on his own.

Once again, we were struggling financially. I decided on top of already working full-time hours to do an extra 12-hour night shift per week at a private hospital in Sydney. My husband took over running the house and chauffeuring the children to their various sporting venues. The shift was 12 hours from 7pm to 7:30am on weekend penalty rates, so the financial hiccough was temporarily solved. I struggled with working so much and making a start on the next stage of interviews for the PhD, but I did what I could to progress my thesis.

The research required me to formulate an extensive literature review and methodology chapter. This immersion into the subject matter provided me with a path for the outline of questions I wanted to ask at this next round of interviews.

I also continued revising my book of fiction and reduced the word count from 158,000 words to 90,000. After receiving enough rejections from traditional publishers to wallpaper my house, I decided to get serious about learning the craft that is fiction writing. This was my one and only escape from the reality of my life — my happy place, the place I never wanted to leave.

At first, when I began working the extra shift at the private hospital I worked on a combined Antenatal/Postnatal Ward. Being a private hospital, the caesarean section rate was very high. It was hard work, with minimal staffing. There was also a nursery made available overnight for mothers who had unsettled babies, which required a staff member to be present at all times if there were babies in the nursery. I worked in the Delivery Suite as well, but as with all private hospitals, a high intervention rate goes hand in hand with services that are underpinned by a medical model. In other words, what the medical officer says, goes. It is fair to say some of those decisions were made to balance other demands on the medical officers' time, such as private practices with patients scheduled to be seen and other hospitals to visit. High intervention rates are the antithesis of nature taking her own course.

This hospital was extremely busy, but unlike the public system, the women were offered an adequate length of time to recover from the birth, were assisted with breast feeding and baby care while receiving good hotel-type service. The service grew exponentially and soon there were only two options; either extend the number of available beds — which takes a good deal of time — or think laterally to come up with an acceptable plan and provide postnatal care for well women and their babies. This was a stroke of brilliance. An entire floor of a local, popular hotel was rented and turned into a four-bed postnatal ward with one midwife on duty. I worked many shifts at this facility. The women loved staying at the hotel because they had double suites in which their husbands and other children could stay with a midwife on hand at all times. The hotel facilities such as the brasserie, the gym and the pool were added bonuses. These were good times and continued on for many months until the extension of the maternity service beds finally reached fruition and were opened.

Soon, I was prepared for the second round of interviews. I had my questions prepared and I was now well informed, thanks to undertaking a comprehensive literature review about whistleblowing, bullying and harassment in nursing. It was time to try and quantify the consequences for each of the nurses as a result of their stories having been made public. As I prepared to meet each of the participants again, I began to worry what effects, dredging up the past would have on them. I researched sensitive studies and tried to understand how the researcher somehow kept themselves safe from the effects of hearing terrible recollections, because it was clear that I would also be affected.

I read a quote by Alfred A. Montapert. I thought on his words for a long time and realised it applied to me and to the other nurses; "Every person has free choice. Free to obey or disobey the Natural Laws. Your choice determines the consequences. Nobody ever did, or ever will, escape the consequences of his choices."

Consequences? What consequences? I wasn't a whistleblower, and neither were my colleagues. We did what was required of us, reporting adverse events and outcomes via the accepted hierarchical channels. How could I have been a nurse for more than thirty years and not know that public reporting of events would be regarded as nonconformity, professional disobedience and a lack of loyalty towards the management structure? This is when I learned that organisational behaviour is inherent and to step outside of that plan is to invoke human nature to punish those who are seen to 'buck the system'.

The irony of this is that the participants and I have been punished for something that we did not do. None of us spoke out publicly. Reporting of sentinel incidents via the established management structure was a professional mandate and a part of our roles. It is when the issue becomes public knowledge that violates the status quo, regardless of the seriousness of the patient outcome or event. I have suffered badly for Narissa's public declarations of adverse outcomes and patient deaths. If my suffering was so extreme, how had the other nurses fared? I thought the guilt from this round of interviews would destroy me.

Monique: Allegations were made against my reputation that I was a drug addict. The Director of Nursing ... said she believed the allegations were true ... she had reported me to the Nurses and Midwives Registration Board. ... Over a period of months ... the waiting ... not knowing if I had a job ... horrible. The Nurses and Midwives Board notified me by mail that the allegations were unfounded and there were no restrictions put on me as a nurse. After I was named in the newspaper article, I took annual leave. Post-traumatic stress syndrome! Fucking oath post-traumatic stress syndrome and no it doesn't go away! That fear factor is there! And it's not far away. It's like 'Oh fuck!' Every so often, it just ignites. It just takes one trigger and you think, 'Fuck here I am again'. In 2004, I had a massive infarct [heart attack] ... and bypass surgery.

Meadhbh: I think primarily the first thing was not sleeping and starting to drink heavily, palpitating, being totally insecure, taking up compulsive eating. Having gone through the compulsive phase to eat, to night sweats, to waking up in a panic, to being somewhere and seeing somebody I perceived to be the General Manager of my hospital which absolutely devastated me to the point where I would have to go home. I stopped going out totally as a result of that. When I had to go to doctors' appointments, I would have to be escorted, because I could not physically do that myself. I stopped looking after the house, didn't cook, didn't shower! [emphasis], lost absolute interest in any kind of self-maintenance. Around that time, my husband left me. I had gone from a size 8 to a size 16 and now I am down to nearly a size 6. I do blame the events at that hospital for the breakup of my marriage.

Violet: I couldn't think. I didn't want to talk. I couldn't think straight. While being a nurse, I picked up staph [a staphylococcus infection]. It never affected me, but with all the stress ... boils ... the pain was excruciating My friends were basically with me every day because at one point I was moribund. It took its toll in the end. I exhausted a couple of friends. At first ... it was all like a fantasy ... I resented the fact that I couldn't do it [commit suicide]. I couldn't ... because I had my son. But there was resentment there because I had to be there for him ... because if I didn't have him, I would be able to get out of this. I hate life ... I hate life. I resent the fact that I have to live life. I wish I wasn't here, but I have to be here for my son. I would give up tomorrow if I could.

Yanaha: Initially I just dropped 10 kilos, couldn't eat ... I shook ... I think part of the weight loss was that I was shaking constantly, my metabolism was in overdrive. That was the most noticeable physical thing. I started to drink ... too much ... [sad laugh]. I was at a point back in 2003, I contemplated jumping from a building ... a very tall building ... but I couldn't get the window open [sad chuckle]. I don't think I really wanted to die ... I just wanted to escape. But yes, psychologically I was as low as I have been ... as low as I would ever, ever want to get. I never want to get to that point again where I felt hopeless.

Simone: The only way I kept going for those four years was ... just to maintain the rage, otherwise I would never have seen it through. I have always responded to stress in a way that is probably not good for my body – overeating, overindulging. In my marriage ... a bitterness ... ultimately took my life in a different direction. And I changed; I was not the same person. I just forgot how to communicate. I can't communicate ... it has destroyed our marriage. The anxiety at night would be overwhelming ... I would have these panic attacks. I never used to drink alcohol, now I drink alcohol. In the first two years, I started gambling. I was going on poker machines and I would be there from almost when it [the club] opened, just sitting there pressing the button. Just pushing it ... a thousand dollars, two thousand dollars, it wouldn't make any difference...

Kathrine: I was severely affected both psychologically and physically by the events at the hospital that employed me as a senior nurse manager. The rage I felt about how I was treated changed me irrevocably; altering my respect for the profession of nursing and the faith I hold for the people I work with. It became obvious; my career at this hospital was over. Little did I realise that reality would be extended to every public hospital in New South Wales for the rest of my nursing career. I now understand post-traumatic stress syndrome. I didn't think I would survive. But I knew the loss of my life would devastate my husband and my children. I couldn't inflict that pain on them ... but some days ... I have been advised by my current employer that because of my perceived whistleblower status, NSW Health will never again employ me in a senior capacity. They have remained true to their word. Today, I have an acute anxiety disorder that will be life-long. The consequence for me and my husband is the loss of a three million dollar investment portfolio that would have seen us comfortable, self-funded retirees at the age of 55. Now we have more than doubled the mortgage, and my husband and I will now have work until we are at least seventy-eight to finally pay off the mortgage. I have learned to fear the fear.

21

After the second round of interviews, I was well and truly rattled when the ever patient darkness extended its black wings and enveloped me again. I didn't know that my colleagues had suffered too. We were all professional nurses who were simply doing our jobs. How did the tables get turned on us and why didn't we see it coming?

The responses to our individual acts of advocacy were not directed to us as nurses, but as individuals, punished with psychological terror, loss of career and financial hardship. Furthermore, we were all left with physical and emotional sequalae that rendered us vulnerable to a lifetime of issues related to substance abuse and addictive behaviours.

All I wanted to do was make their pain go away. They didn't deserve to be punished; they deserved congratulations from the profession and public alike. In conducting the interviews, I felt like I was deliberately setting out to hurt them. Oh God. The guilt was smothering.

Monique: Ah, well … sometimes I cried (after the interviews). I have just had to accept and leave the shit where it belongs, it doesn't belong with me … but it is a scar, and when you look at a scar, you remember how you got it and that it will never go away.

Meadhbh: I am very willing to go through this process with you [being a participant in the interviews] but, it scares the bejesus out of me, because it [the fear] is coming back, often. I mean I do feel choked up about it. I know the last time after you left, I was wired. And that is not a criticism of you; it was talking about things that I had locked away. I don't think it is ever going to go away. It's always going to be there. Suddenly Pandora's Box is open and I actually feel … I physically feel myself droop. You know when you are in that semi-foetal position, it is like you want to protect your head, because you are going to get beaten. I felt beaten by them, physically beaten.

Violet: When you have got depression, it takes every second of every minute of every day of every week to just move on to just get through the next second, the next minute and the next day.

Yanaha: The whole experience is something that I just wanted to put to bed, it is difficult … I just don't want to go there anymore.

Simone: Oh, it has been really hard [crying]. That last one [the second interview] … you know I think it is good in a way [to verbalise], because it is really easy to push this down and to pretend everything is fine and go on. But you can't do something like this and say that it hasn't affected you.

I relived my experience over and over and over again while the narratives of my colleagues hammered me like a hail of bricks! I totally underestimated what it means to be a participant observer in research. The interviews were extremely difficult because I knew the nurses of this study professionally, and some I knew socially. For me it was the double whammy! I relived my experience ... not just once, but each time we met for the interviews and again and again when I revisited the transcripts. I felt like a masochist, wanting ... needing ... to hear and record the stories, while at the same time witnessing the pain and the suffering. I was terrified I would invoke some recollection or reaction from the past that would harm them, because in truth, they would never have offered anyone else the raw accounts of the experiences that they offered to me. The acute anxiety disorder I developed during my own whistleblower experience roared to life not only when we met for the interviews, but again and again when I went through the narratives during the writing of my thesis. I thought the second round of the interviews and the subsequent write-up would kill me.

I was frightened by the effect the interview questions were having on the nurses. I had always been a nurturer and unconsciously, I developed an overwhelming need to protect my participants. It was hideous to witness the distress of these women. I couldn't stand it. I felt like a sadist, deliberately and knowingly inflicting distress by encouraging them to speak about their past and dredge up their demons. What I didn't realise then, was, the greater their distress, the more I subconsciously narrowed my level of inquiry.

This research experience presented an enormous contradiction for me; the need to understand the experiences of the nurses and my need to ensure they were treated fairly and came to no harm by resurrection of these events. I fell victim to the trap of the participant observer. I lost my way and struggled with self-loathing, knowing that I was contributing to their pain and hardship. All I wanted was for the world to know what it is for an Australian nurse/midwife to be labelled as a whistleblower. And here I was, learning the greatest lesson of all - no pain no gain; and it sickened me.

By then, I thought I understood the challenges of 'sensitive research' and its potential for harm. Christ, I totally underestimated the transfer of feelings, emotions and the reactions of life-altering events from the nurses who had experienced the phenomena, to me, the researcher. I also underestimated the potential for this qualitative research to harm me, because their stories and my story, were the same. Exposure to their pain and recollections significantly increased a resurgence of painful memories in my personal, stuck-in-top-gear thought loupe which reignited and incited my darkest fears.

My research supervisors, correctly identified my challenge in the development of an appropriate scholarly scope of inquiry for the study; a scope that embraced the wider world experience of whistleblowing. Many times, unconsciously, my protectionist interpretations had devolved the study into what was an exposé of, and was limited to, the experiences of the six nurses involved in the research. Their pain became my pain and the focus of the study became narrowed and flawed, not by intent but by my need to understand how six professional, highly qualified and skilled nurses, in the course of executing their various roles, could be, like me, lost to nursing and made lifelong professional pariahs.

My supervisors understood how I had become sidetracked. They gave me strategies on how to move forward and how to expand and correct the direction of the thesis. In some ways, it was a relief to expand my range of thinking from my singular focus to widening the thought boundaries to include experiences elsewhere, out there in the world.

In 2008, by virtue of my own experiences and the experiences of my colleagues, I saw nursing and the New South Wales Department of Health through very different eyes. After the numerous hearings and Inquiries into the state of health in New South Wales, the findings of Peter Garling SC, into The Special Commission of Inquiry into Acute Care Services in NSW Public Hospitals were released. The full transcript of the hearing can be found here:

https://www.cec.health.nsw.gov.au/__data/assets/pdf_file/0011/258698/Garling-Inquiry.pdf.

I was impressed by this man right from the beginning. No questions were too hard and he was serious in his endeavour to discover what it was that ailed this public hospital system. To gain this quantum of knowledge, he did the unthinkable, he created a communication channel and consulted with hundreds of clinicians and front-line public hospital staff. I was surprised when I encountered the online link and naturally, contributed to the study. Of course, I had plenty to say about the state of health in New South Wales, far more than the link and text box allowed for on the Health Intranet.

Ages later, I received an invitation to participate in the New South Wales Health Complaints Commission (HCCC) at the behest of Peter Garling QC. It seems he took the time to read my submission and combined with his own investigations, believed that as a health provider, the state of New South Wales was in big trouble.

In 2009, I was appointed as an Expert Reviewer for the Health Complaints Commission in matters of midwifery. It was a role I enjoyed immensely, sifting through boxes and boxes of evidence, putting together the pieces of the puzzle to ascertain what had gone wrong during a woman's labour or birth; how that event could have been predicted or prevented, and what best practice principles should be applied in the future. Irony really is a strange bed fellow.

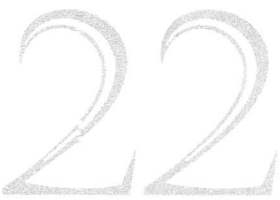

22

Maybe I will forever be naïve. The powerlessness of the individual clinicians was what really concerned me. If managers choose to not act upon information given to them about patient safety or patient outcomes, what is the nurse to do? Sure, the clinician can go up the next rung of the management ladder with their concerns, but that is a step for the fool hardy, as the local manager would potentially be viewed as not doing their job properly. Secondly, moving concerns up the ladder puts the clinician in the unenviable position of appearing to have little faith in the local management, while upper management can be potentially resentful about the ball being passed into their court, forcing their hand to either address the issue or become complicit in deliberate ignorance. For clinicians, reporting of incidents of concern is fodder for conflict; for there is a fine line between truth telling and whistleblowing. So, few see the big picture where issues of concern should invoke investigation, best practice principles and resolution for an improved patient journey in the future.

Garling QC's findings reflected what we as nurses had tried to address:

• Engagement of clinicians to address recruitment and retention issues.

• Implementation in substantial change in clinical governance and how problems are reported and addressed.

• Address of the 'clinician - manager' divide.

• Address of the loss of accountability in hospitals since the abolition of area health service boards.

• The public health system needs injection of additional funding to 'pull it back from the brink.'

• Better partnership between the state and federal governments.

And there it was… In six succinct points; unfortunately, all too late for us. But at least by our declarations and subsequent public appearances, our substantiated claims of the failure of intra-institutional structures, or poor self-regulation and governance, error reporting and investigation had been accepted as truth. Clinical governance structures had now become part of the institution of health care in New South Wales. I am so proud of this outcome. As individuals, we achieved what we had set out to do. We had all advocated for patients and as a result, in a convoluted way, health care became safer - albeit years later.

Garling QC's findings and recommendations, was a hell of a wake-up call for New South Wales Health. This major public utility that was voracious in its spending of hard-earned tax payers' dollars had been exposed not only to the state that it served but also nationally and internationally as an organisation that fostered a culture of nondisclosure and cover up. There was nowhere to hide. The multitude of investigations and Inquires resulted in a call for redemption from the senior managers of the health service. The CEO of the hospital where I worked and reported Monique's findings to, lost his job, while the General Manager who intimidated Meadhbh and Yanaha resigned in a deal to be offered a $165,000AU position with another area health service.

Reports reveal Narissa was 'warned off' by the then area health service chairman who regaled all of the nurses labelled as whistleblowers as having psychiatric issues. He was eventually forced to stand down. Despite the findings of Garling QC, just three weeks before the state election and after three months of deliberation, the Health Commission Complaints Commission handed down its findings, that there were no questions to be answered and no cover-ups.

Nurses from this area health service watched helplessly as the media showcased the whistleblower nurses being sidelined, marginalised and victimised with their jobs on the line. Other nurses who by virtue of the fact that they were employed by these two hospitals were abused publicly, spat on and berated by the general public, just for being nurses that worked in the hospitals that were splashed across the news.

A former nurse took the helm of the HCCC and before the official report could be tabled, one of Sydney's biggest tabloids spelled out the horrible truth that at least 17 patients (of a total 47 complaints), had died after receiving unsafe, inadequate or questionable care at the two hospitals. But not one individual, be they medical officer, nurse or hospital administrator, was named, blamed or held accountable for the litany of tragedies.

Due to NSW Health's poor track record of transparency and disclosure, Garling QC's findings supported the establishment of an Incident Information Management System (IIMS). It was established as a key component to linking adverse patient outcomes and safety issues with the reporting of problems. The program was computer based - which was problematic in itself, as the average age of registered nurses and midwives in New South Wales was over forty, with a good number being baby boomers, a mass exodus of which are getting ready to retire.

Hospitals had introduced local Intranets whereby policies and procedures were posted and newsletters from the area health service were available online for staff. The lack of technological expertise was not such an issue. If there was an article of interest, hard copies could be printed. Not so with the IIMS, it was an online reporting mechanism, whereby data was gathered regarding patient safety issues from which the factors could be analysed and provided as the foundation for system wide quality improvements.

I was particularly proud when the IIMs was first introduced because it meant every employee, be they the CEO, a medical officer, a domestic attendant or a gardener could report adverse events, outcomes and near misses. Each report was appointed a Severity Access Code from 1-4. A SAC 1 being the most serious and a SAC 3 or 4 being an incident requiring local action by local managers.

However, instead of using the IIMS as a positive service improvement tool, too often it was used as a punitive vehicle of complaint from one worker about another. Over time, health workers lost faith in the IIMS system as a negative report about a colleague meant an interview with the local manager, threat with the Code of Conduct and possible disciplinary consequences without the issue ever being fully and truthfully explored. The other problem with the IIMs was that the responsibility for address of all notifications that had a SAC of 3 or 4 were the responsibility of the local manager. It seems a good many of those reports never came to light and were never addressed. Perhaps they were filed in the delete bin. In Health, no one airs their dirty laundry in public and gets away with it. No one.

This was a time in my life when I just put one foot in front of the other, kept working, sleeping, eating and living the life of a disconnected person. The only time I was truly happy was when I was writing. My first book was now published What a journey. I had learned the hard truth that writing a book IS. NOT. EASY.

Since that time, I have learned a good deal about what it takes to capture a reader's attention for long enough to consider purchasing the book. I have also learned that the writing is perhaps the easiest part, it is the accumulation of a talented team of artists responsible for promotion, marketing, editing, formatting and the creation of 'jump off the shelves' covers that requires commitment, continuity and the end product - creation of a brand that is uniquely mine.

Writing the words was then, and continues to be, cathartic for me. The characters in my books became my family while I engross myself in a world that I love, so removed from my real world, the one I didn't want to participate in.

In Australia, the concept of mateship is an inherent part of being an Aussie; no doubt a legacy from our great, great convict grandparents that has become an entrenched part of the Australian psyche. We are a free, open and friendly race.

There is a story that Bill and Hilary Clinton were walking along a beach in north Queensland, followed by a sea of black suits with ear wigs, when a local fisherman tipped his hat and said, "Mornin" Bill, mornin' Hill. We're havin' a Barbee over at my place tonight. Drop by if you have the time."

With that, he picked up his bucket and fishing rod and headed towards his house. I am not sure whether this story is just urban legend or whether in fact it did happen. But the story does capture the free-living spirit that is quintessentially Australian.

The Australian colloquial term 'you don't do in a mate' hailed from our humble beginnings and heavily influences the Australian work ethic - after all, if one convict got the lash, all in the group got the lash. The canon of mateship continues to exist today and is absolute; with the expectation that workers do not 'dob' to the suits (management) for any reason. Another expectation of the Australian work ethic is that organisations will step up and 'do the right thing'. Mateship, camaraderie and transparency of moral behaviour by organisations, combined with a cultural aversion to 'dobbers' are expectations of Australian workers. That being said, does the act of public disclosure exact harsher reactions and punishments for Australian whistleblowers? A bloody good question.

23

The labelling of my colleagues and I as having pre-existing mental health issues is cited in the research as classic bullying behaviour; intended to cloud the issue at hand by shifting the point of focus to the person(s) who have made the allegations. Logic confirms, if the person who raised the concern is mad, then there is no issue, just a figment of a troubled mind. Nurses who speak out are viewed as troublemakers and are likewise punished. In order to keep their jobs, they are often required by the employer to undergo psychiatric assessment. This action is twofold. Firstly, in order to discredit the nurse, a formal diagnosis is gained, confirming some form of mental discourse that would provide an 'acceptable' explanation for the nurse's actions or allegations. The second function of this form of enforced psychiatric evaluation is to completely destroy the nurse's credibility for any future disclosures. After all, who believes the ravings of a mad person?

From personal experience, I have reason to believe that there are psychiatrists on the payroll of the public health system that are handsomely remunerated to hand down findings in favour of Health. Alternatively, if a nurse seeks compensation for psychiatric trauma incurred during a whistleblowing event, the nurse will be found to be completely sane and in no way damaged by the events he or she was involved in. For nurses who make allegations about the public health system, it is a lose/lose situation.

Nursing is not just an eight-hour-a-day job. The nature of the work shapes character by exposure to extreme human experiences, from birth to death. The qualities of compassion, empathy and advocacy are expected traits of a professional nurse/midwife. These inherent characteristics are the foundation for the promotion of truth and the protection of patients from harm. Nurses are called upon to be accountable to the patient, and yet nurses' have little legitimate power within the healthcare system.

The demand for ethical practice places the nurse in a most precarious position; for at what point, does advocacy become whistleblowing? Why should there ever be an occasion when a nurse, to advocate for a patient, must speak out beyond the management structures of the employing organisation? When is the level of advocacy enough? Does the concept of advocacy have a ceiling of acceptability? My experience leads me to believe that it does, and if a nurse steps beyond that fine line of acceptability, the nurse will be sanctioned, vilified and professionally ruined.

The nurses in my PhD study collectively shared more than 200 years of clinical and professional experience. As senior nurses, we were all aware of the expected line of hierarchical reporting and the protocols associated with raising awareness of adverse outcomes or issues of patient safety; processes enacted by each of us; with the same outcome - no action by those to whom the events were reported. Yet, by virtue of the fact that our experiences became public due to Narissa's declarations, we were targeted by the media and labelled as whistleblower nurses. A very cruel lesson indeed. Exposure by the media destroyed reputations as professional nurses who were guilty of nothing more than advocating for their patients.

Meadhbh: I went through all of the channels, including the union and nobody would listen. So I don't truly see myself as a whistleblower.

Simone: [Whistleblower] I have hated the term. In fact, if I see it in regards to anything I think I don't want to be in the club — thanks! I don't want to be in the club … All I ever wanted to do was to do my job. I never set out to do anything except do my job…

Violet: I don't see myself as it [a whistleblower] … I just see myself as [long pause] as someone who told the truth, who was morally and ethically correct and told the truth…

Yanaha: I have never been comfortable with that ... label ... the definition of a whistleblower, I think, is somebody working in their professional environment who sees open corruption, that sort of thing and goes public with the information. Which isn't how I saw our situation ... I still don't understand it. 'Cause all I did in my view was what I was supposed to do. I alerted my seniors to concerns that I had about the clinical competence of another healthcare professional, and I ended up losing my job because of it.

Monique: I have done nothing wrong. I have done the right thing and I am the one that had to leave.

Kathrine: How could I have been labelled a whistleblower when escalation of a situation likely to invoke the interest of the media was part of my job description?

By this time, I imagine we all hoped H. G. Wells really had created a time machine from which we could all go back and redo the past few years. Yet we are all career nurses. If we could all go back to prior to the year 2000, would we make the same professional choices?

Monique: I would make the same choices. But I wouldn't trust the system. I kicked myself afterwards. I think I should have gone home and rung the police that night and told them that I was confident that the patient had died in suspicious circumstances … but made it anonymously. I did do it again. That night you were on [Kathrine on duty as an After-Hours Manager]. You protected another patient … I remember you saying to the ICU nurse that you would be making sure that her death was not expedited by drug orders from the ICU doctor. She was dying, but not fast enough for him! But she did die of natural causes. That is what nursing is to me. I can still see the husband of that lady sitting by her bedside waiting for her to die. [In the future] I would do it different. But I would never not say anything.

Meadhbh: I don't have the same faith in people that I had. And maybe my faith was naive. I never believed that there were people out there who would set out to destroy somebody. I mean in politics yeah, that is what they do. I am more selective about what I would say and what I would do around people. I choose my friends very carefully now, which can be very isolating. But yeah, I believe I am much more cautious and wary … if I sense there is a surgeon … and I am aware that there are problems … I ain't goin' there again. I am very clear I ain't goin' there again, because emotionally and physically I just couldn't deal with it. And yes, it is the ostrich with its head in the sand, but it is time for somebody else to do it. I will never put myself on the line again.

Violet: Yeah. I would do it again … because you have to. Not that anyone is telling you that you have to. You have to do the right thing. It is like us when we look at murderers and we ask how could you live with yourself after you have murdered someone. You are hiding something … not doing the right thing.

Yanaha: I would. Absolutely I would … I know that. I would be the first person to speak out. I won't stand by and watch a patient being harmed. I would, because I have to … it is some intrinsic law in me maybe and I guess that is why I don't want to ever again come across it.

Simone: I love my job and I know that I am very well respected in my job. I still love it, I still have a passion for it, I still believe it is for me, but I guess it is like a marriage … I love it, but I am not in love with it anymore and when you are not in love anymore you just go through the motions … But the thing that burdens me the most … is that if only I could go back a bit and change some of the things and the way that we did them, we would have been more successful. Because ultimately it is a game … and you know you have to be on top of the game.

Kathrine: Yes. Speaking out was never optional for me. In the future, I will still speak out however I will pick my battles and be better prepared to deal with unsupportive managers and systems that don't protect truth tellers. I regret unwittingly being drawn into Narissa's often hysterical and grossly exaggerated agenda against public hospitals in New South Wales. By virtue of both of us being employed by the same Area Health Service it was easy for the media to align me with her and the other participants as a rogue vigilante group of whistleblower nurses. Nothing could have been further from the truth.

In hindsight, I now know I am exactly the sort of nurse who becomes labelled as a whistleblower; I expect high standards of care, honesty and integrity. My whistleblower colleagues, the participants in this study, are nurses who shared the same standards. Our lives have been eternally, personally and professionally, altered as a result of being labelled whistleblowers by the media and by our peers. Against these personal blows, as advocates for our patients, we demonstrated our commitment to quality patient care.

The Inquiries into patient care within the two hospitals identified by the nurses in this research proved to be a watershed for change in public health in the state of New South Wales. By virtue of publicly exposing adverse patient outcomes and raising patient safety issues, we were instrumental in the establishment of clinical governance structures within healthcare in the state of New South Wales. Our efforts were not wasted.

As is the way with scandal, it reaches its flashpoint then dies out. After a long time, the government lost interest in us. Via the media, the public were vigorously reassured by NSW Health that all of the issues brought to light by Narissa had been addressed, and that patients were back in safe hands; a new guard was in place. The media side show finally died down. We were no longer front-page news and the journalists had moved on to the next tragedy from which they could sensationalise heartbreak and despair. I sometimes wonder how those people sleep at night, knowing their stories will damage reputations or, as in our case, cause lifelong damage.

On reflection, there were some good outcomes from our participation in the various Inquiries that would go a long way to protect the people of New South Wales in the future. But what about us? What about our futures?

Monique: Oh … I just take every day as it comes. I am surviving [working as an agency nurse] and at the moment, I am happy…

Meadhbh: I want out of nursing [working as a clinician] … I am the educator for the operating theatre at a private hospital in Sydney. I am looking at doing the Cert IV [Certificate 4 Training and Assessment] with a view to going to do some training in the universities. I am working with students now and I am running the peri-operative course.

Yanaha: Working in a private hospital I am selective about the surgeons that I will work with. There are still things going on all the time. My strategy [chuckle] is to not be where those things are. I intend to continue working until I am about 65 — not full time. I intend to work full time until I am about 60, and then probably part time for another five years and then … walk away.

Violet: I will never nurse again and the reason being is because of the way that they [management] turned [on me]. I don't believe that I would ever be able to work without them looking to be able to find a problem.

Simone: I feel disassociated from my colleagues ... I feel very much that I am no longer part of the ranks. [Now working as an enrolled nurse in operating theatres in a major tertiary referral hospital]. I would have to say first, ostracisation ... I felt totally ostracised [as a consequence of speaking out].

Kathrine: After being informed that NSW Health has imposed a lifetime veto upon me preventing me from ever again being appointed to a senior nursing position within the New South Wales public health system, I honestly didn't think I would ever recover from the loss of my career. That blow has proven to be true. The void in my life left me, for years, empty and sad.

It took a simple turn of events to help me to see that a successful future was still possible, albeit down a far different path from the one I ever imagined. I had written my first book of fiction, which has been assessed as having high commercial probability. If my book sells and writing becomes a viable option, I will walk away from nursing forever to become a full-time author. In this case, the pen may indeed prove mightier than the sword.

To be labelled as a whistleblower is usually a once-in-a-lifetime event. Even though we did not deliberately put ourselves under the media spotlight, the outcomes of raising our individual issues of concern were far from expected. I have learned that whistleblowing, regardless of how the information became public, is never regarded as trifling and the blame for wrong doing is reversed onto the person(s) who spoke out.

Nursing is cited in the literature as promoting the highest degree of workplace bullying and harassment of any profession. The New South Wales Health Department, in recognition of this fact, has promoted a Zero Tolerance Policy along with workplace training about bullying and harassment, which is little more than lip service to a significant workforce problem. There is a proven link between bullying of Australian nurses and the current recruitment and retention crisis in the nursing workforce.

Bullying and harassment of nurses, regardless of the spruiking of New South Wales Health is workplace violence that is not addressed. This lack of address of an extreme workplace issue is a constant threat to every nurse in this state. However, being bullied as a nurse is a far cry from how perceived whistleblower nurses are treated. The effect of speaking out is not limited to the workplace, the ripple effect extended into personal and social lives. Fair play? Absolutely not. How can actions in the workplace spill-over into personal and private lives? The answer is, they shouldn't, but they do.

Monique: Oh yeah, when I had to take time off work ... financial ... yeah — very much. I don't think any amount of money would undo what has been done to me. Initially for my family at first it was a little bit of embarrassment ... The allegations ... the drug allegations and all that sort of thing ... where they actually mentioned my name ... I think they were proud of me ... I think they are still proud of me ... My mom ... not so much ... you know saying 'You were stupid,' but in a way even though she wouldn't say anything, I think she is proud of me. Whenever I go to work, she says, 'Now behave yourself' [laughing]. She still to this day says, 'Behave yourself'!

Meadhbh: Look, no there were not financial [losses], but financial is of no value to me, money has no value. It was the loss of myself and the absolute destruction of my marriage and the subsequent consequences for my children and none of us have recovered from that really. My son had only been married about three months when my husband left. He moved in here with his wife. They were really supportive to me and helped me get through it. But for the first year of their marriage, they were dealing with the consequences of the breakup of my marriage of thirty odd years ... My son of twenty-nine won't even acknowledge his father exists. My daughter came back from overseas and I had to deal with my kids crying on Father's Day. I do blame the hospital that employed me, because I know I became someone different to who I was. I mean obviously, it [the hospital] on its own didn't cause it [the marriage break-up], but it certainly pushed the boat out. My husband ... my ex ... would tell you it was my obsession with that hospital and my lack of interest in him, my home, myself, all of those things that arose from this, because he saw no end to it.

Violet: Financially ... big ... I lost my job, I lost my career, my future and my superannuation... so my security and independence. I lived off my savings for a year and then I had to go on a pension for the first time in my life and I never thought I would. I don't speak to my family, so I can't speak about that ... except for my son. It is awful when your son has to look after you at such a young age and sees you crying ... to wake up one day on the lounge room floor crying and your son has curled up asleep on the floor next to you ... Our whole lifestyle has changed. I am not the same person ... You lose complete trust. I don't trust anyone. I don't believe in anyone ... I used to believe ... God will look after those who deserve it, but it doesn't happen. My whole belief system has changed actually. My psych [psychiatrist] said that was the day that I stopped believing in people. And I believe that to be true.

Yanaha: Financially ... well I was compensated. I was lucky. I think Meadhbh and I were both extremely lucky because our case came to a head right at the height of everything and the Department of Health was very keen to put it to bed. They were very keen to settle ... I try not to talk about it too much, because I don't want to bore people and I don't want it to be the sum total of who I am, and after a while, no matter what the disaster is that has happened, people do get sick of hearing about it. I think they do, and I try to remind myself, 'Now don't talk about it because people are sick of hearing about it! Put it to bed!'

Simone: Financial ... it is really difficult to quantify because it was very untimely; my husband became retrenched at the same time, so it is very hard to put a money value on it. If you sat down and wrote it all out, I got paid out eighty-nine thousand dollars plus legal expenses, so it was about one hundred and ten thousand dollars. Now I have this house and it is mortgaged to the maximum ... there is nothing left. The eighty thousand I got paid out ... I had had no wage for two years; I had borrowed from my father forty thousand dollars. The other forty thousand, I had some on credit cards, bills and things like that. So from a financial point of view ... we have estimated that it has probably cost us one hundred thousand dollars. It changed my identity really. My husband says I am not the same person, and our marriage has suffered greatly — greatly. I don't know that it won't be over ... My daughter said to me one day, 'Why did you have to be a whistleblower nurse? Why did you have to do that? Why couldn't you just let one of those other people do that? Why did my Mom have to do that? Why couldn't you just be my Mum?' [sobbing]

Kathrine: Absolutely! In order to receive the monies owed to me, I was forced by the Area Health Service lawyers to sign a waiver that guaranteed I would never bring a lawsuit against the service. I received poor legal advice and signed the waiver. My wage as a senior nurse manager was halved when I was forced to accept a clinical position. My mortgage of course was brokered on my original income. As a consequence, I have for years now had two jobs. I work full time night duty as a midwife and my second job is at a private hospital working one twelve-hour night shift a week. So, fifty-two hours a week, every week, to ensure the bank didn't foreclose on my home. Of course, the investment portfolio was an enormous loss, not only in terms of the change to our retirement plans, but in the accumulation of significantly more debt to get out of those contracts. My husband and I attempted once to calculate the financial losses, including the loss of the properties, income and additional interest paid because of increased mortgages. We stopped calculating when we got to about three million dollars, which is somewhere near what we will be out of pocket by the time I retire — which, God willing, will be well into my seventies. As for my family, they have stood by me and are proud that I told the truth. However, they understand first-hand what it is to be a whistleblower and what it is to suffer because of it. It is sad when children comprehend that kind of suffering. As for socially, when something like this happens, it doesn't take long to figure out who your friends are.

It was some time after the flashlights stopped popping that we became old news. The health service had been exposed as having seriously flawed safety, investigative processes and reporting mechanisms. The whistleblower nurses, although not intentionally, had their fifteen minutes of fame and were rewarded with significant career, financial and personal losses.

It was Narissa who was forever tenacious, empowered with the strength of ten lions who contacted each of us to advise she had been contacted by a Sydney law firm who specialised in medical negligence. She encouraged us (with the exception of Monique, who was unknown to her) to contact the law firm and bring a class action against the Area Health Service for our losses. We followed Narissa's lead and in due time, we were contacted by the law firm and evidence was collected with a view to litigation. Several months into the evidence collection stage, the law firm advised they were no longer in a position where to represent us as they had accepted another contract which presented a conflict of interest for our collective claim. As is the way with lawyers, they will always back the party most likely to win. In this case they crossed the floor to represent the Area Health Service!

Until this time, at no stage did we ever consider a collective legal 'fight back' attempt, because we were never a group in the first instance. Rather, each nurse sought individual representation independent of each other. This lack of group 'action' is testimony to our innocence and just how beaten we were. A collective action could have been a powerful choice, but clear, appropriate decision-making was not possible for any of us; it was challenge enough to get up in the morning and face another day of uncertainty and fear.

As they say, life goes on but for me I now know this platitude; instead of meaning life goes on in a good and positive way, means the sun will continue to come up and go down. Nothing more, nothing less. The world will carry on about its business and as nurses we were on the scrap heap and yesterday's news. But, what of me? I am a lifer, nursing as a career is really all that I know. I started nursing training in April 1975, just two months after I turned seventeen, which was the minimum age for course entry at that time. After everything that had happened to me and at my stage of life, I didn't have the energy or the drive to consider embarking upon more study to create a new direction and a new career path. I have always been a nurse, but after an event such as I had just experienced, I was a very different nurse. How could I continue in a career with a profession that had turned its back on me? How could I still feel an obligation to advocate for patients to keep them safe, when advocation had almost destroyed me?

I felt isolated, marginalised and discarded as unwanted. I was like a blind person, shuffling and feeling my way forward, trying to grasp hold of familiar things. As a nurse/midwife, I knew my life would never be the same. My colleagues, likewise, realised that we were all personally and professionally changed. The final round of interviews confirmed what I knew to be true. To continue to work as a nurse (or not), each of my colleagues had come to the realisation that a plan for the future was required to keep each of us safe for the rest of our working lives. There were decisions to be made about our professional futures and how each of us as individuals would achieve that end.

Monique: [Laughing] By choosing to be an agency nurse! That's it! I am doing what I love. I like that because before, when I was working full time at a Sydney hospital, I was going to the same ward and the same shit! But now, I am not permanent. Nuh! The politics and the sweeping under the carpet – Nuh! This way I can do what I love until I can't do it anymore, but still nurse the way I was taught to nurse.

Meadhbh: The bottom line for me is that I want out of nursing! Yes, I want out of the [public] hospital system and spend my time thinking about what I am going to do. At the moment I am [working in a private hospital operating theatre], just starting Certificate IV and I am hoping with my experience as an educator in theatre that I will be able to get in somewhere to do some teaching. But there is no way I am continuing in the [public] hospital system.

Violet: I am too afraid to be autonomous. I did try and go back at one point when I thought I was getting better ... I went to agency nursing ... I lasted five shifts and I was a mess. I couldn't concentrate, you know all the symptoms were there ... in the end I froze on my last shift. I came in on a night shift ... I can't even remember what was wrong with him [the patient] ... he arrested [cardiac arrest] towards the end of my shift and I had to give adrenaline. I rushed to the cart and got the adrenaline and I couldn't give it. I couldn't give it and I threw it at the nurse on the other side of the bed and said, 'You give it' and I stood back. At the end of that the supervisor said, 'Do you want to go home?' I said yes and I left and didn't even ask for my pay. That was when I knew I would never be a nurse again ... I am ashamed.

Yanaha: Now, I am guarded. I am very guarded with any situation that is any way out of the normal ... I used to be a multi-skilled perioperative nurse. Now I have narrowed my focus to just orthopaedic surgery because it is safe! I don't work with anaesthetists. I don't work with any other surgeons ... this is a way of protecting myself ... I have to stay in my own little world.

Simone: As an endorsed enrolled nurse working in theatre I cannulate, I take blood, I give drugs, I assist in massive procedures ... I give blood. I do it all, not the anaesthetist who checks the drugs, I intubate I think that within my own mind, I will practice in a safe manner, being taught by professionals ... and that I do so to a safe level, that will not harm the patient and that I am educated ... I will not do any more than that ... and at times it will exceed what the hospital thinks I should be allowed to do, what you think I should be allowed to do, what the Nurses Registration Board thinks I am allowed to do. We all exceed our scope of practice; we are all capable of exceeding our scope of practice. And the only reason it is not universal is because we are not all capable, but most nurses are — particularly when they have been nursing for a long time.

Kathrine: Safe? Absolutely I needed to make sure I was safe! People are afraid of me. Experience has taught me to be paranoid and to be highly defensive in my practice now. Since becoming a clinician, I have been brutally targeted in the workplace, and because I am unrepentant, they [middle and upper management] continue to target me. Interestingly, since the management of the hospital became aware of the subject matter of my research and its soon-to-be-completed status, I have been left blessedly alone. I need to keep *me* safe — I may not survive another experience like this. To keep myself safe, I ensure there is a paper trail of everything I do. Any conflict I diarise, any unusual events, I document voluminously in the patient record and again diarise. If we have difficult patients, I ensure my conversations are witnessed by a colleague, with countersigned documentation in the patient record. I leave nothing to chance now.

After 18 months, the research interviews were finally completed and we all went our separate ways. To this day I am saddened by the loss of Violet, Meadhbh, Monique and Yanaha to the public hospital system and that Simone, to survive, has had to find a workplace where she can be safe. Patients need nurses who are strong advocates to ensure care and safety standards are maintained. But nurses are mere flesh and blood. In the end, we all must choose our own road into the future.

The blessed peace fiction writing gave me was a God-send. It brought with it a very welcome distraction from the fear and anxiety I continued to experience while working as a nurse/midwife. After the second full rewrite of my book, I had a chance meeting with a woman who worked at our local supermarket. I was soon to learn she had five books published and was working slavishly on titles to come. She is a highly competent and experienced writer who is well informed regarding the 'rules' of fiction writing.

My friend was very generous in the sharing her time and her knowledge. There was just one problem; I think like a nurse, so my writing style was technical, in terms of language and descriptions. I cannot recall the number of times my friend would make a most unladylike snort, roll her eyes and say, 'Oh God, there she is again, nurse Kathrine and her bloody nursing textbook!'

The second issue with my writing style was that, after so many years of academic writing which is in narrative style, my know-it-all friend would ask me, 'Who the hell is speaking in this scene? Is this dialogue coming from the Gods?"

No. I was guilty of using omniscient voice - that is to say a third-person narrator. This, in contemporary fiction, is apparently a mortal sin. It seems one must literally get into the mind of the character and be that character - called Deep Point of View, which presents all sorts of conundrums.

Who knew there were so many rules to writing fiction. My book had been revised too many times to count. I thought Warrior Born: Book 1 of the Katana Series (written under the pseudonym of Kathrine Leannan) was a good story but hey, my opinion was hardly unbiased. With great trepidation, I gave the manuscript to my friend for review and guidance. When the work came back to me about three weeks later, the pages looked like a mortally wounded soldier. Her sabre sharp, red pen had slashed my work of brilliance to pieces. Seriously? Did she not know this story was my baby? I was deflated and curled up metaphorically in the foetal position and thought very mean things about her and her brutal red pen.

This was completely new ground for me. I was not used to being a green newbie! It took a while (with me all the while kicking and screaming), but eventually I stopped being a diva and got over myself. I would learn this craft and all of its bloody rules or I would die in the attempt. I could do this! For crying out loud, I held four degrees with a fifth imminent and am an intelligent human being. No amount of learning could have prepared me for what was to come.

Lesson One: works of fiction are not children. They are like any other product that is produced for sale.

Lesson Two: the ability to stand back and be objective is imperative.

Lesson Three: constructive criticism is not personal (even if it feels like it is).

Lesson Four: readers do not want to read a nursing text book. Sure, they love to read about all the drama and the blood and the guts, but not in clinical language; otherwise, the mind pictures do not form and the reader will never connect with the story or the author.

Lesson Five: the hardest for me to grasp and develop - stop writing in the narrative and write in the voice, thoughts, actions of the character. I learned from my smart-arse friend that I was the queen of 'head hopping'... er... what? There is a golden rule (yes, another one) - one scene - one character. Of course, there can be many characters in a scene but the scene belongs to only one, that way the reader experiences what the character experiences in his/her interactions with others. This is where the visceral descriptors of taste, smell, touch and feelings come alive on the page.

Easier said than done. But be damned if it was going to beat me.

Writing was my escape. When I was with my characters, I was happy and I was safe. I continued to exasperate my friend who persisted in drilling the rules of good fiction writing into my brain. Life became easier, because for a few hours of each day I could be the person I was before the whistleblowing event, the me who saw beauty in Autumn leaves and the goodness in people. I recall the times outside of my writing escapes as being monotonous and lonely. My husband and I became mates with my writing mentor and her husband. It was good to have friends again. They are good people.

They say it takes a village to raise a child. Likewise, it also takes a team of talented people to produce a marketable book. In 2014 I was offered a three-book contract from a traditional publisher and my book was published. I had done it! I had written a book that was now out there for posterity. I laugh every time I recall my brother's face after he turned the last page. Shocked he said, "God Kath, it's like a real book!"

I continued to work full-time as a night duty midwife and when the postnatal hotel service wound down, I worked on the maternity ward there for a while. But when I observed an Enrolled Nurses working out of her professional scope of practice and medical officers performing brutal deliveries, I had to walk away. In the past I would never have done that. My entrenched sense of advocacy, to do the right thing would have forced me to document events and seek improvements. However, in a facility that was driven by a medical model - that is whatever the medical officer says, goes, there is little scope for change. I cannot condone unprofessional practice. I had learned the hard way to pick my battles. Not my fight - walk away.

In 2016, after six gruelling years of interviews and heart-breaking research, I graduated from the University of New England in beautiful Armidale in rural New South Wales as a Doctor of Philosophy. I will be forever grateful to my colleagues for their truths. I doubt they would have been so forthcoming with someone who didn't know what they had been through.

At work, I rightfully began to use the title of medical officer in documented medical records. As is my habit, after completing the documentation, I place my signature which was followed by RN., RM., PhD. Probably three months after I began documenting this way, I was advised formally via the internal mail that as I am a nurse, I am not entitled to use the title of Doctor, as it is confusing.

The documentation of my nursing qualifications at the completion of each entry into patient records clearly identifies the professional source of the research. The academic testamur I produced to confirm the acquisition of a PhD, clearly entitled me to use the title of Doctor. Professional ignorance is a pervasive and destructive thing. I had worked hard to achieve the PhD and be damned if I was going to curtail to the demand by executive nurses, that as a nurse, I was not to use the title. I consulted with the university who confirmed my entitlement. I then met with management to advise them of my intention to continue to use the title. I know, I know, call me petty, but I just couldn't help but give them a little insight into the history of the title. A doctorate is awarded to a person who has successfully completed a degree that is composed entirely of research. The use of the term Doctor for medical practitioners, history offered courtesy use of the title because of the position they held in society, whether they held a doctoral academic qualification of not. I am entitled to use the title Doctor by virtue of the fact that I have earned it.

Management, both middle and upper, became gun shy of me, which is hardly surprising, given that my PhD is primarily about bullying and harassment in the nursing profession. The fact that I am articulate and have a strong social conscience made me a problem. This was particularly true for the newly appointed Senior Nurse Manager of Women's Services. She had come from a hospital not too far away with little to no experience and a reputation that preceded her. In her case the Peter Principle certainly applied. We were not going to be friends.

By now dear readers, you will have gleaned that I take patient safety very seriously. I cannot recount the number of times I submitted risk management reports of women walking from the Postnatal Ward to the Antenatal Ward beverage area carrying their baby under one arm, while holding a polystyrene cup in the other, filled with boiling water. Often, there would be a trail of spilled liquid on the floor for some hapless soul to slip. Not to mention the risk of burns and scalds to either the mother or the baby is too high to even begin to calculate. Just imagine the headlines: 'Newborn Baby is Critical Condition After Being Scalded by Hot Water at Hospital X.' That would certainly sell some papers.

In response to my numerous incident reports about this very matter, I was advised that it was a woman's right to walk around with her baby and to do as she pleases. I was further advised I did not have the right to interfere in the process. The right? No, a professional responsibility.

How could I observe such risky practices and not intervene? Time after time, I asked women at the beverage bay if they would like me to hold the baby, or if I could make the drink and carry it back to her bed.

It was on spilled liquid outside the beverage bay, that ironically, I slipped and fell. I incurred a full thickness tear to the meniscus (cartilage) of my left knee which required me to work in a full knee brace (it takes A LOT before nurses and midwives abandon shifts as recrimination and criticism is common). Today, this injury greatly affects my ability to manage stairs and has contributed to numerous falls.

There was a clear lack of commonsense and leadership in this Division and risk management did not take a high priority.

One night I came to work to find floor-to-ceiling sheets of thick plastic draped down the walls. The air reeked and all of the desks and equipment at the Nurses Station were covered in a thick layer of white particulate dust. It seemed the two wards were to be repainted. Instead of decanting and painting one ward at a time, the decision was made to paint around the patients and their babies. Clearly the directive was to get the painting done as quick as possible; as evidenced by the hapless fly that had been painted over on the back of the staff toilet door of the Antenatal Ward.

Not long after the shift started, my eyes started to swell as red blotches broke out wherever the dust had settled on my skin. My airways and sinuses were burning and I was a mess. I went home and took several of photographs of the reaction my body was having and rang WorkCover the next morning. WorkCover is the Australian workplace health and safety regulator. An investigation was undertaken and the Division was forced to enact safety measures to protect patients and staff. Unfortunately for me, it was all a little too late.

The executive of the hospital did not believe I had incurred an allergic reaction to the particulate paint matter. To accept that fact is to also accept responsibility for any/all ongoing health issues caused by the exposure. My Dermatologist confirmed I had incurred a severe allergic reaction to the paint dust. I remember asking him, "What happens the next time I am exposed to paint dust?" His answer, "Possible anaphylaxis. We will just have to wait and see."

I saw babies with paint dust on their bunny rugs and cots and the furniture in the inhabited rooms was likewise heavily contaminated. How many of those babies would have developed allergies to paint dust in the future after such extreme exposure?

So now, I had experienced two serious workplace injuries that have both proven to cause lifelong consequences for me - falls and acute sinusitis that until this time I had never experienced; requiring supervision by an Ear Nose and Throat Specialist and daily medication to control the symptoms. So much for risk management. An oxymoron at this hospital if ever there was one.

Middle managers such as Nursing Unit Managers are in a very difficult position. They are the quintessential meat in the sandwich. While they want to support their staff, if they wish to survive in the position, they often become puppets for the level of management above. This can be a good thing in that, less experienced managers can be mentored and grow both personally and professionally. That was not the way of things in this case. My local manager, who had once been my friend, had very little choice in what she did. I regret the loss of contact with her and her friendship. She was a good person and midwife with a kind heart. She became another victim of poor leadership and harassment.

The service started to unravel at the seams under the 'leadership' of the Senior Nurse Manager. She was a bully who demanded compliance. Dissension grew in the ranks. When the Level 2 Nursery was closed, I knew this foolish decision was just the tip of the iceberg under the current leadership. The divide between the two wards continued to grow and innovation was dead. It was work, work, work - get those women out and free up the beds. The sanctity of quality midwifery care was violated before our very eyes. It was bedlam. If there was an empty bed then a patient went into it. It didn't matter that the patient was for a Prostin induction and the bed was on the Postnatal Ward with midwives who had next to no contemporaneous experience in caring for labouring women. Likewise, it didn't matter if a patient, recovering from complex gynaecological surgery, was located beside a postnatal woman with an unsettled, crying baby. Bums in beds was all that mattered. Job satisfaction for me had withered and died.

The increasing tensions for this service caused me to feel agitated and unsafe - for very good reason. The acuity of the patients didn't match the availability of registered midwives. The ceiling was lifted on the number of Prostin inductions that could be booked each day. The restriction had been imposed on the booking process in the first instance, to avoid this very situation – too many patients and not enough midwives to keep them safe. The new Senior Nurse Manager was very keen to get the medical officers on side, so the flood gates were thrown open – come one, come all – no restrictions on the number of bookings for Prostin, Cervagem or elective Caesarean section patients. The medical officers were delighted but the midwives were run ragged and no one cared.

Nurses and midwives have to think on their feet. It is a quality that is necessary in an ever-changing patient environment. The antenatal midwives on the afternoon shift developed protectionist strategies for themselves by either delaying the commencement of scheduled Prostin inductions or request a medical officer come to the ward and insert the Prostin. I understand why this happened; no one wants to be put in a situation where a baby is delivered in a bed in the ward because the midwife had too many patients to care for and too little time to devote to a labouring woman. If a baby did deliver on the ward, there was always blame and shame appointed to the midwife for not getting the patient to the Delivery Suite in time.

I will admit, I was terrified to go to work, but I was damned if I was going to be caught up in another adverse patient outcome because my concerns fell on deaf ears. By now, dear reader, you must be thinking that I am a masochist and question why the hell I didn't just resign and walk away. It's a valid question and the answer is simple; at 50-something, I had given my entire adult life to nursing and midwifery. I would do everything possible to ensure patients did not come to harm and after all I had been through, how could I walk away? If I didn't speak up, then who the hell would?

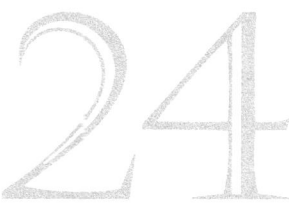

24

My husband and I discussed the issues at this hospital endlessly as the tendrils of darkness reached out to me again. I recognised the feelings, the abrupt change in mood and the accelerated rate of my thoughts. I recited my mantra until I felt the strength to say enough, I reject the cloak of depression and fear that does its darndest to consume me. I was working in an environment of deliberate ignorance of practice and safety issues. I needed to stay safe so I began to collect evidence that the workplace was derelict in its duty to investigate issues of patient concern and patient safety.

Over the years, I had submitted numerous IIMS reports outlining my concerns regarding staffing, skill mix, patient acuity and near misses to the local management. I continued that practice as it created a paper trail. I got nothing in return except criticism with trumped up accusations of poor performance and abdication of responsibility in the nursing care I offer to patients; none of which could be substantiated, but there were no apologies forthcoming. In the end, I realised that no matter how often I reported these issues, no action was going to be taken. To acknowledge these issues would mean complex investigations and so, it was easier to simply ignore the extreme risks to patients and file them away under the ravings of a mad woman.

The raft of reports I submitted went into cyber space, never to be seen or heard about again. I used to joke that there was a black hole between the IIMs send button and the management email inboxes. Nevertheless, the risks existed and continued.

I have always maintained and supported due process. In my days of university lecturing, I impressed upon my students the meaning of advocacy and the onerous responsibility that goes along with it. I instilled in them the correct way in which to raise and report issues of concern or events that involve patient safety. Professional behaviour includes accountability and reporting. There is a professional hierarchy of reporting that includes the appropriate channels to address concerns. I have always believed it to be imperative that local issues are solved with local solutions by the people who do the job. If these parameters are not met, the issue, in my experience, will not stay solved. In my case however, there were no solutions forthcoming, because no one wanted to know.

I knew the clock was ticking. This was familiar ground for me. I had been here before and I was just about at the end of my tolerance. As far as I was concerned, this workplace was an accident waiting to happen and it was only a matter of time until it did. The fear was growing, not only for me, but also for my colleagues. The workload situation was becoming untenable and none of us wanted to be caught up in the misery of an adverse patient outcome. The solution for this organisation was to make it personal, appoint blame and not follow up on incidents. The fault was always with the employee.

I was doing the right thing which was always important to me. I was reporting, but nothing was happening. I felt frustrated and tired of being a reasonable and professional nurse; the one who escalated her concerns and trusted in the willingness and indeed capacity of the management of the service to step up and do the right thing. I depended upon them, and so did my patients. We were deluded.

It was 2016 and I was Dr Kathrine Grover. I had been erroneously labelled a whistleblower. I had done my darndest to bring to light my issues of concern and I had reached the end of the line. I recall this moment as if it were yesterday. I emailed the Director of Nursing and the General Manager of my concerns and of my repeated attempts to have these issues addressed.

By now, I journalised everything I did at work and that documentation became the backbone of my submission to the executive of the hospital. By this point, I had no issue with being labelled as a whistleblower, for those who speak out, blow the whistle, call it what you will, are just trying to do the right thing when every other avenue of reporting has been denied to me. I am no longer insulted by the term whistleblower, because I am a staunch patient advocate and proud of it.

I knew what had to be done and I felt I had nothing to lose. I itemised my concerns as a list of demands, that, if not met by close-of-business on the date of my nomination, I would go to the media and expose the risks I was aware of, that had long gone unaddressed. I was called to meet with two senior executives and I laid my cards on the table. I provided evidence of risk management reporting and unactioned submitted IIIMS. I made it crystal clear that I would go through with my threat to go to the media and my subsequent connections with senior journalists. I was not prepared to wait any longer for a patient to come to harm. My neck was on the chopping block, but I didn't care. I would do the right thing for how could I continue to work there and do nothing? Time to do what I do best – solve potentially risk-laden processes for patient, whatever it takes.

Nothing mobilised the management of Health like the threat of media exposure. Suddenly, there were innumerable investigations and the spotlight was on the Senior Nurse Manager of the Division. I was called to speak with the Director of Nursing on a few occasions and felt satisfied that the wheels of justice were indeed in motion and that due process would reveal that there were major issues to be addressed. Life seemed to take on a rhythmic pace and for a while, I believed the organisation would rise up and take ownership of the issues requiring improvement. I felt a kind of peace and hope that life could just get back to some semblance of normal, where I could work night shift on the Antenatal Ward with a team of 'regulars' whom I enjoyed working with and whom I trusted.

I have never really considered the true meaning of the word 'catalyst'. I certainly have a very good understanding of it now. One night shift, I was in charge when a patient was to be downgraded from the Intensive Care Unit to the Postnatal Ward. They had several empty beds and had the capacity to accept the patient. I received a call from the Team Leader of the Intensive Care Unit to say the patient had been refused by the Postnatal Ward and therefore would come to the last remaining bed on the Antenatal Ward. I contacted the (relieving) After-Hours Manager who confirmed the patient had been refused by the Team Leader of the Postnatal Ward. I reminded her that no patient could be refused admission to the Postnatal Ward if there is capacity to accept them. She agreed and intimated the patient was of an acuity level that would be better met on the Antenatal Ward. I accepted the patient, but not the argument.

I discussed the matter with the Team Leader, who said the ICU patient was 'too sick' to come to the Postnatal Ward, despite having several empty beds and more staff on the Antenatal Ward. I informed the Team Leader that the patient would fill our only remaining bed on the Antenatal Ward. As a matter of professional courtesy, I advised her that I would submit a report based on the refusal of the patient because undoubtedly, the event would feature in the After-Hours Managers report to the Director of Nursing. As it turned out, the patient was complicated and required one-on-one nursing care which meant the other midwife and the non-endorsed enrolled nurse on duty on the Antenatal Ward had the other twenty-three patients to care for. I cared for the ICU patient. She was stabilised without incident; we got through the shift and the patient was on the mend.

The very next night, I was informed a delegation of staff from the Postnatal Ward had gone to speak with the Senior Nurse Manager after completion of their shift. She apparently gave them their five minutes of fame and listened empathetically to how busy they were and why they couldn't have accepted the patient. She then questioned them specifically about me - about my clinical skills and my professional practice. It was reported to me that they had stated they relied on me when I was on duty for professional support and guidance. As an expert clinician, they stated they were always glad when I was on duty. The Senior Nurse Manager wasn't happy. She wasn't getting the answers she wanted, until one of the midwives declared that there were times when I did my writing at work...

A colleague gave me the 'heads up' about the covert meeting with the Senior Nurse Manager. That afternoon, she was in the tea room listening to a boasting session by the postnatal staff involved in the patient refusal incident. About how they told the Senior Nurse Manager all about my other life as an author. I wasn't surprised that they would try to explain their point of view to the Senior Nurse Manager, they were afraid of her intimidatory, condescending behaviour.

I listened to the information and took the news in my stride. Until that is, my colleague informed me that the focus of the discussion was not patient related, but concerned me and my writing. Eureka! She now had the evidence. She garnered sworn, signed statements from the staff who met with her to discredit me. I was trouble for her and she meant to get rid of me.

The Director of Nursing and the General Manager took my threat to go to the media seriously. The wheels of motion were well in play and the Senior Nurse Manager was suddenly under considerable scrutiny. To her, based on the number of complaints I had submitted, I was the thorn in her side that had brought the spotlight down upon her.

Sometime later, the Senior Nurse Manager played her hand. I received a letter accusing me of fraudulent behaviour. Allegedly I wrote numerous books - a saleable product, making thousands of dollars while on paid time by the health service. Yes, I did write books and yes, I wish I made thousands of dollars in sales but I never made a secret of my writing, nor did I ever deny it. My colleagues equally kept themselves busy on quiet nights with reading or craft. One colleague, a budding professional photographer, processed her photo shoots during quiet periods. Where was the distinction? The distinction lay in the fact that it was my name on the IIMS and to save their own skins, the postnatal staff had given the Senior Nurse Manager all the ammunition she needed to discredit me and detract the focus from her.

This was an incredibly tense and unpleasant time.

I came to work one night and one of my colleagues appeared withdrawn. Eventually, she said, "I don't know if I should tell you this or not. But if it happened to me, I know you'd tell me."

I suddenly had that dead, sinking feeling in my gut and the next few minutes went into slow motion. I could hear the words my colleague was speaking and I could see her mouth moving, but everything around me was blurred. There was just me and her words that got sucked into a vortex of fear and decompensation. It was no doubt, an awkward moment for my colleague. She told me that the Senior Nurse Manager had unexpectedly arrived to work at around 5am on my days off to interview staff about me as a clinician and as someone who wrote books for personal gain at work. Everyone I worked with was well aware that I was an author. The Senior Nurse Manager, was also, very aware of my history as a nurse advocate.

Rather than be verbally demanding, she was supportive to the staff in her quest for damaging evidence about me. The Senior Nurse Manager sympathetically portrayed abhorrence that I would increase my colleague's workloads by shirking my professional responsibilities to selfishly write books instead of attending to patient care. Several of the staff took the bait like marlin and ran with it - never miss an opportunity to get in good with the boss. All the staff interviewed were informed they were professionally bound to silence and that the conversations she had undertaken with them were to be held in the strictest of confidence, otherwise they would be disciplined and held in breach of the Code of Conduct. It is my view that the Code of Conduct has become a weapon used as a threat against nurses and midwives when issues arise requiring explanation. Definitely time for a rethink.

The Senior Nurse Manager, like a cat with a struggling mouse in its mouth stood tall and dropped the bombshell at the feet of the Director of Nursing and the General Manager. It seemed they had made an error; she was not the problem, I was. She needed to divert the spotlight from herself and her actions were nothing more than an act of subterfuge and quiet malice.

For me, the world stopped. I struggled to stay out of the place of darkness, but it was a near thing. The difference with this experience was that the divisive actions of the Senior Nurse Manager were not only lodged against my professional integrity, but also against me, the person.

I spoke with the Director of Nursing who was unaware of the interrogation tactics that had been used by the Senior Nurse Manager. She agreed that I should take a period of leave and to return to work the workplace would be adding fuel to a deliberately set fire. This was a very challenging time for me. A violation of trust had occurred so I worried endlessly about how I could ever work with long term colleagues who had so readily stabbed me in the back.

The Director of Nursing encouraged me to lodge a complaint against the Senior Nurse Manager. I did so but should have known there would be another agenda at play. All hell broke loose and once again, my life took a different direction.

I stayed at home and questioned why I had become a nurse in the first place. I mean seriously, the worst thing that could happen to me if I were a Marine Biologist would be that I could be eaten by a shark or poisoned by a lethal cephalopod. At least the death would be reasonable, given the line of work. I, however, was filled with self-doubt and distrust for everyone around me. I had become very un-me, a person I didn't like at all. My husband was my pillar, my strength, my safety net. However, you don't live a life with a person like me, who had experienced so much, and not be affected. My dark enemy depression, wound herself around his thoughts until he too, was sad. He also worked in Health and because of 10 years of saturation with disturbing events and abuse, he too, had become suspicious and distrusting of those around him, which continues today. I will forever regret that such a happy, gregarious man could know and understand first-hand that place where I go when the darkness finds me. It terrified me to the point where we had to make a pact that only one of us could devolve into the darkness at a time. One must be the sentinel to make sure the other returns to reality. It was a tough call, but so are we.

I was contacted several times by the Director of Nursing whom I knew feared I would end my own life. I was grateful for her concern. I was also aware that if I did in fact choose to leave this mortal coil, my husband would expose my death as a consequence of being a nurse in a violent, poorly managed organisation whose leaders hid behind truths rather than have the public know what a bloody disgrace the place truly was. He also knew my senior journalist contact details and if I perished, between them, no one would be left standing. I am not a vindictive person but it was comforting to know that the truth would be exposed about patient safety and adverse outcomes and my death would have been a result of doing the right thing.

I starting seeing another psychologist who was a seasoned clinician who had been involved in debriefing and supporting workers where there had been deaths on worksites. He also had worked with policemen who had seen too much of the evil of life that their minds could no longer function. I wasn't the first nurse whose stories he had heard. I told him all of my truths and he believed me. He asked me outright, "Do you intend to kill yourself?"

I remember the pause and the absolute quiet in the room. "Yes, I have considered it. The peace on the other side would be amazing."

I let the peace and quiet be replaced with images of my family. I am the glue and the universe put me here to help others. So no, I didn't want to be dead. I wanted to find peace.

How could I make the long journey back to a place where I no longer cringed in fear of what would happen next, or stop being vulnerable to the words and actions of others? Was that even possible, given how altered I was compared to the enthusiastic, assertive nurse I had once been? How had the warrior become a victim? Time is an insidious, erosive shaper of perception that feeds on experiences and emotion. I was like a sky driver who had spent 40 years in free fall, being buffeted and thrown off course by the power players in Health. But, be damned if I was going to hit the ground.

As is the way of things, when a staff member is unable to work because of perceived psychological distress, they are assigned a Return-to-Work coordinator from the Department of Human Resources. A file is created and evidence is collected. During this process, I was required to see a Psychiatrist to evaluate firstly whether or not I was telling the truth, and secondly to confirm or deny the existence and/or depth of psychological distress. His report confirmed I was suffering from severe psychological distress that was workplace related. His recommendation was that I did not return to the Antenatal Ward. His report also confirmed suicidal ideation.

I continued to have contact with the Return-to-Work personnel which, I now realise, was really just a tick box exercise; all the boxes must be duly ticked in case there is an extreme adverse outcome, like suicide. The subsequent investigation would conclude all had been done for the hapless worker.

After a long time, the Director of Nursing encouraged me to return to work. Not to the front line, but to a position well away from the hospital. I thought this was an ideal choice to ease me back into the workforce, although I think unconsciously the survivor in me had already ruled out return to the clinical area as a midwife, ever again.

I was employed in an odd sort of thrown together position in a Community Health Centre. This was not only a new beginning for me, it was a completely new experience as I had never worked in Community Health and really had no understanding of what community nurses did. My policy and procedure writing skills came to the fore and I met some really great people, two of which I am still friends with to this day. We worked well together as a team and I experienced a different side of health that was proactive, instead of reactive.

The management of chronic disease in the community is a challenge for all health providers with our aging population. This team was buoyant, energetic and focussed on getting the job done. It was good to be among young nurses again, to experience their energy and enthusiasm. There was one manager who deliberately targeted one of the team members, seemingly to vent her frustrations. As is the way with bullies, the most vulnerable targets give the greatest satisfaction. I witnessed my colleague's distress and supported her with strategies to manage the bully and to depersonalise the cutting remarks. Like a younger me, my colleague would take on criticism as a personal insult, only in this case it was personal. She struggled to disassociate the feelings from office politics. I like to think I had a positive effect on her ability to keep things in perspective. It is all too easy to become hurt by intentionally spiteful words or accusations. It takes a considerable amount of maturity to toughen up to the harsh world of nursing. Like I have always said to the students whom I have taught at university and to all the young nurses I have encountered who struggle with the bully girls - "It's not personal! Shields up!"

I was really enjoying my time at the Community Health Centre. I had next to no contact with any of the other midwives or Nurses I had worked with as a Clinician; with the exception of one Enrolled Nurse who is now and will always be a very decent human being and a loyal friend. C. is one of those people whom only the very lucky meet, because she is dependable, supportive and as constant as the crash of waves on the shore.

My energy levels were returning and I was looking toward a brighter future in nursing. I had reconciled myself to the fact that to survive I could not and would not return to the clinical front line. It was at this time that I acknowledged I was forever broken and like all broken things, they must be handled with care. I had by this time accepted that it was okay to acknowledge I was broken, even though deep down, the warrior in me struggled with the dents in my armour.

The Director of Nursing checked in with me every so often. I advised her of my acceptance of my brokenness and in the interests of my mental health I was not going to return to the clinical workplace as that would not be in my best interests. She advised me of the investigations that had been conducted regarding the Senior Nurse Manager and requested I meet with the investigation team to discuss my concerns. This meeting was conducted in the office of my Clinical Psychologist. I guess they thought this to be the best place given that I had emphatically declared to the Director of Nursing that I was done with this life. The investigators were very empathetic and made copious notes. After the interview was over, I was hopeful that a positive outcome would result for the patients and staff of the maternity service.

Some weeks later, I met with the Director of Nursing and the Return-to-Work representative from Human Resources. I advised them that I was not prepared to return to the Antenatal Ward based on the risk it posed to me. I was informed that I would be required to attend a nominated Psychiatrist again for an evaluation. I attended the interview. It was the same Psychiatrist I had seen months before and explained what had transpired over the past few months and of my decision and reasons for not wanting to return to the antenatal ward. This meeting couldn't have been more different from the last. Gone was the empathetic, caring professional. In front of me sat a person who agreed I had been through a tough time, but that was now in the past. It was time to move forward - no real harm done, carry on. No matter how hard I tried to impress upon him the inherent dangers to myself if I returned to that environment, he was having no part of it. Case closed.

I arrived to work one morning at the Community Health Centre with a head full of ideas about process improvement, Australian benchmarks and Best Practice Principles when I was informed my time at the Community Health Centre was over.

Management had been informed I was not damaged by the events on the Antenatal ward and that I was required to return to my substantive position. I rang and spoke to the Return-to-Work representative assigned to my case to try and gain some understanding of this decision. She advised a meeting would be set up with my employer and a plan to return to the antenatal ward would be discussed.

I went to the meeting to discuss my future as a Midwife employed at that hospital. During the course of the conversation, I was advised the Senior Nurse Manager of the maternity service had been on extended leave, this absence was to enable a review of my submitted complaints and evidence. A thorough investigation had been held, including ransacking her office to find years of complaints that had not been responded to. It was too late to act on any of those matters. The conclusion drawn was what I already knew to be true, that the Peter Principle applied. The Senior Nurse Manager did not have the experience or the education to execute such a senior role. My allegations about her failure to act upon unsafe issues were proven. Likewise, her attempt to collect covert damaging information about me was proven to be unfounded and the allegations against me were dismissed. The Senior Nurse Manager was removed from the position.

I was told the Senior Nurse Manager was no longer employed by the health service and would never be employed by them again. The last I heard; she was working for a nursing agency. I was requested to return to my substantive role or to any other ward within the Maternity service. My throat began to close up and the walls started to come in. I heard myself speak, but I don't know how I managed to utter the words. I advised I no longer had the strength to face the ever-present issues on a night-to-night basis. I had done my tours. I had nothing left to give. That was when the real truth behind the support offered to me and the granted extended paid leave fell into place.

The Health Service, thanks to my constant concern for patient safety had achieved its desired outcome. The Senior Nurse Manager was found to be guilty of non-address of complaints, of professional behaviour breeches and well... a mess. However, in Health it is very difficult to get people out of their positions. There has to be a major breach in the Code of Conduct, fraud or criminal activity for a person to lose their job, even then the person may only be shifted sideways but continue to be employed. In my efforts to raise awareness of patient safety, staffing and skill mix issues, I had unwittingly played right into the hands of the Executives of the hospital who were aware she was a problem but had no real way to address her poor work performance.

After it was proven that the Senior Nurse Manager had skulked around and interrogated staff, the Area Health Service now had due cause to step in and address the problem. The fact that I had admitted to suicidal ideation gave them more impetus to go after this woman - and they did. She became a casualty of her own ego and poor skills and was removed from the position. I don't regret what I did in raising the issues, nor does she have my sympathy. In my mind justice was served.

The Senior Nurse Manager was gone, so the problem was solved. The Psychiatrist's report stated I had fully recovered and was not suffering from depression, nor were there any issues of concern that would prohibit me from returning to my substantive position. I discussed this finding with my psychologist who was well acquainted with the Psychiatrist in question. He made no attempt to hide his disgust as he recounted other cases reviewed by this particular Psychiatrist who always found in favour of the employer - thanks to the significant fees attached to clear organisations of any responsibility.

I was at a crossroads with only two possibilities for the future - either return to work as a Midwife or not. The Director of Nursing asked me if I had considered retirement. I remember being shocked and a little insulted at the question. That was a defining moment for me. Without saying so, she was suggesting I leave my job. She knew just how low I had been. I also know that thanks to the shonky Psychiatrist's report, that the Health Service was only obliged to reinstate me to my substantive position.

Going back to working on the Antenatal ward wasn't an option. Returning to the Community Health Service also wasn't an option as in real terms the position I held there was a Return-to-Work position, not a funded position. It became apparent I had outlived my usefulness. The end game had been achieved. The Senior Nurse Manager was gone. I remember after the meeting, pulling out of the car park and waiting at the lights to turn onto the road towards home. I was suddenly overwhelmed by a tsunami of unexpected, overwhelming relief. I felt so light, I could have floated out of the window of the car, which is the exact opposite of what I thought I should have been feeling. I felt free, like a prisoner, released after serving a life time sentence.

I did indeed walk away. I resigned. There was no fanfare, no farewell dinner, no gifts and no good wishes. All of which was fitting. I don't regret my actions. I have been a Nurse all of my adult life. Once a Nurse, always a Nurse. It is like a second skin that is never shed. This was probably one of the worst financial decisions I have ever made. I withdrew the maximum amount of non-preserved, accessible funds from my Superannuation which I estimated would pay me a wage and fund the mortgage for the next 18 months or so. For the first time in my life, I didn't have a plan.

The life lessons I learned during this time taught me to know which battles are mine and which are not. I no longer feel compelled to be the champion of all causes. My Dad was right to teach me to 'do the right thing'. What I have learned is to 'do the right thing if the responsibility is mine to do so.'

25

I soon discovered that I am not good at sitting at home, being idle. In 2016 I was enjoying lunch with a colleague who shared similar opinions and is patient-centric in her approach to service delivery. She was a Senior Manager of a Community Health Service. She is a human dynamo with endless energy and is an all-round good woman. After a couple of glasses of Sauvignon Blanc, she suggested I apply for a job at the facility where she was the manager with view to being her heir apparent as she was considering retirement. At first, I thought she was joking, but then I realised she was deadly serious as high standards of patient care were as important to her as they are to me. She realised she could retire and be reassured she was handing over the reins to someone of a like ilk.

The job, to get a foot in the door and to have the opportunity to 'learn the business' was a telehealth position for a registered nurse where, after two weeks orientation to the role, I could have remote access and work from home. The actual service was about two and a half hours drive from where I live. My colleague, who was now my senior manager agreed if I was required to come to the Centre, I would work a six-hour day with the other two hours paid travelling time.

I applied for a job as a Registered Nurse and was called to interview. I got the job and looked forward to working as a nurse again and being productive. The training for the role to my very great surprise was problematic, as was the intake process for patients as the process was not generic. Rather, the five main referral sources of patients to community services, had service specific intake procedures. Human nature being what it is, the propensity for error at the point of intake was high. These errors were a source of significant tension between the Intake Centre and the five Community Health services. For registered nurses in my role, there was no definitive training program for new employees. Rather, it was on the job training, sitting next to a clinician, listening to their responses to the patient, which was completely redundant given that the patient side of the conversation could not be heard. This type of induction equated to the quintessential learn by your mistake's paradigm. As a high achiever who takes pride in my work, this was an unacceptable learning methodology because if the registered nurses didn't get the intake right, the knock-on effect was delay in the patient receiving services.

I have never had much tolerance for rudeness and unprofessional behaviour. I travelled to and from this facility every day for three weeks, working the agreed hours. Sydney traffic is bedlam and I lived 65kms away. The travelling was a killer and in no way sustainable. If I got home two hours after finishing work, I considered I had done well. It was exhausting. At the conclusion of the two weeks orientation, it was clear to me, and I imagine everyone else, that I was not ready to work unsupported in a remote location by working at home. I requested another week extension.

I don't believe I have ever experienced such chaos. I sought to understand why these intake processes that were so prone to human error were not replaced with a generic intake paradigm. It soon became clear that professional territorialism, resistance and resentment was the answer to the question. The Community Health services themselves had operated independently for years. They referred and cross-referred patients and kept their own houses in order. When the centralised Intake Centre was established, all of the referrals came in via that service, after the patient was admitted they were then referred on to the services in the community.

For years, the us and them mentality had flourished. If an admission error was made by an Intake Centre staff member, the error was escalated by Community Health Managers to high-level senior managers. This was petty, petulant behaviour that was did nothing but continue to erode the relationships. It was in my view, the constant criticism, embarrassment and ridicule incurred by the Intake Centre was central to the collateral damage that occurred as a result. Rather than cop the inevitable barrage of complaint and stress, the nursing Team Leader and the senior administration staff member checked every referral before they went live to the relevant services. Honestly, the utilisation of two senior staff members to act as sniffer dogs for errors, to me, screams dysfunction process. However, I digress...

There is no amount of money in the world that would cause me to covet the Team Leader's job. What I witnessed of her every day work experience was professionally abhorrent. As in medieval times, like being flayed - constantly gouging the same raw, exact spot; as a constant stream of abuse and criticism ate away at her self-confidence and fed her stress levels to breaking point. She was reactive and took her frustrations and anger out on the staff employed at the Intake Centre. I do not believe she was a bully by nature. I believe she was pushed everyday beyond the point of reason.

On the Friday of the third week of working at the Intake Centre, my colleague announced I would be working from home, starting from the following Monday. I will never forget the look on the Team Leader's face. It was absolute astonishment. The message her eyes conveyed to me were, "You are in no way ready to work from home."

I could see her steeling herself for all of the errors I was going to make with the intakes I did from home. She knew it and I knew it. I was just not ready to work unsupported.

I stuffed up so many times. I was constantly in tears. The Team Leader in the beginning tried to be supportive, but in the end, she was like a crow tearing at the flesh of carrion.

My anxiety levels were though the roof. It was decided that I would come into the Intake Centre one day a week, which I thought was a logical and good suggestion. However, by this stage the Team Leader despised me and the feeling was likewise. I would cringe when she would scream across the room to some poor staff member, "If you want to work here, you have to be tough enough to take it!"

Floods of tears were a daily occurrence from various staff members. It was when staff member declared to me that she had commenced taking antidepressants to cope with the abuse from the Team Leader and the job that I knew I was not just over thinking her behaviour. At the end of one shift the Team Leader was abusive towards me and never being one to step back from a fight, I went home and emailed a complaint about her to my colleague and the Operations Manager.

After a meeting with my colleague, I discussed my observations to date and the highly problematic intake process. The Team Leader and I agreed we could work together in a professional manner. My mistake was not taking up my colleague's offer to escalate the complaint to Human Resources. After a few months, my colleague announced she had set the date to begin her well-earned retirement. By that time, she too realised the knowledge gap in the induction of new staff needed to be closed. She arranged for the Team Leader and I to work on a guide for the induction of new employees. It was a good experience as the Team Leader had worked at the Intake Centre for years. She had a considerable amount corporate knowledge, albeit to date currently undocumented and unshared that would be very beneficial to newbies.

After my colleague retired, a senior manager who was also my colleague from the hospital where I worked as the Delivery Suite Manager stepped up into the role in an acting capacity. It was at that point that everything that had been agreed to by my colleague i.e. that I continue as a remote worker with the exception of when required to attend the Intake Centre for training or education sessions. That agreement went out the window the moment my colleague was out the door. The Operations Manager and the Team Leader claimed no knowledge of these agreed working conditions, despite the fact that I had been working these hours for the past six months. I was informed (threatened) by the

Operations Manager that she could insist I work all of my shifts at the Intake Centre. What could I do? I was foolish enough not to have insisted my original terms of employment be documented and signed off. All I had was an agreement of the hours I would work when participating in the Intake Guide for new staff members - which reflected the exact agreed arrangements. When I raised this, I was informed those criteria of employment were specific to that project and were now null and void.

My shifts working at the Intake Centre increased from one to three days per week. So, eight and a half hours worked plus a total of five hours of travelling time per day - thirteen and a half hour days, back-to-back; that is if I actually left on time. The Team Leader was brutal to anyone who packed up at the end of their shift and went home. She liked to clear the board of all the intakes and staff were expected to stay on their own time. Of course, the organisational stance was that no one is expected to work past their end of shift time. Or the one that used to really rile me was no one was permitted to work overtime unless it is authorised by the Team Leader or the Operations Manager. So, guess what? It was either cop a barrage of abuse from the Team Leader for having the audacity to leave work at the completion of the shift or keep your head down and just keep working, keep working, keep working on your own time. There was never any sign off for overtime.

I hated working at the Intake Centre. In fact, I hated the job altogether because the Team Leader projected her stress levels onto me and all the other staff working there. She was like a pressure cooker, screaming and abusing others was her release valve. I remember one staff member who was regularly in tears, but who was also afraid of the Team Leader. I heard her whisper that she was going to record one of the Team Leader's rants and upload it onto YouTube. I encouraged her not to do that as she would lose her job and the problem - the Team Leader would still be there. I should have just shut up and let her do it.

I went on annual leave to Townsville to visit my Mom. I was depressed and PTSD threatened to kick back in again. I was determined and confident that I had the skills now to ensure that place of darkness never over took my life ever again. I honestly was not sure if I devolved into the mire of profound depression again, that I would make it back to normality again. I decided that when I returned to Sydney, I would get another job and resign from the Intake Centre.

The best laid plans of mice and men.

After I returned from leave, I spoke once again to the Operations Manager about my intolerance of the bullying and harassing tactics of the Team Leader. I advised I had made up my mind that I could no longer work productively with her. I also advised of my intention to resign after I secured a new job. The Operations Manager arranged a meeting with the Team Leader and myself. The outcome was that the Team Leader was incredulous that she was the reason for my resignation. The Operations Manager by this stage was in a situation that was well and truly above her experience level, so, when in doubt, do nothing. Not long after this meeting, the situation came to a head. Late one shift the Team Leader asked me to do an intake, which I did. She then asked me to do another. I advised her it was ten minutes until it was shifting finish time and I was not able to stay back. I began packing up my equipment when she demanded. "What do you think you're doing?"

I advised my shift was finished and I was going home. She sneered at me, "You can go home when I tell you it is time to go home."

A flash of rage filled me I collected my bags, said goodnight to the other remaining staff member, ignored the Team Leader and left the building. On the way home, I ran off the road and caused a chaotic situation for myself and at least four other cars. It was my fault; I wasn't concentrating on driving. I was concentrating on how the hell I was going to survive working with the Team Leader until I secured a new position.

I was absolutely shaken when I got home. I burst into tears and the look on my poor husband's face said it all, Jesus, she's going to fall off her twig again. He was right, the darkness awaited me. I went and saw my GP and his advice was for once in my life, to put myself first and get out of the Intake Centre. He had been with me all the other times when depression and darkness overtook me.

I am an idiot. I should have just resigned and walked away. I wrote a letter of complaint accusing the Team Leader of bullying and harassment. When will I ever learn? There is no truth or transparency in NSW Health if the managers concerned choose not to uphold it. The matter went to Human Resources who never contacted me to discuss my concerns. A meeting was organised by the Operations Manager with the Team Leader present. To those who know HR etiquette it will be clear that this suggestion was a highly inappropriate way to address this issue. I contacted the New South Wales Nurses and Midwives Association who advised me to consider carefully my decision about attending this meeting. I refused the invitation to attend as there was clear risk to my mental health.

For the second time in my life, I did something I swore I would never do, I resigned without a job to go to and walked away. Nothing was resolved but I was out of there. Those issues were not mine to solve. It was maybe a year later I was contacted by an Intake Staff member who was a particular whipping person for the Team Leader. She asked me to put my case forward to a Board member whose name she gave as she needed support for her particular fight at this workplace of nightmares. I did nothing. I grappled with it, but I did nothing. Finally, I had learned the lesson. Is it my fight? No, walk away.

It is now two four years since I resigned. That decision was financially reckless but correct for my health and wellbeing. I have applied for at least 50 jobs since that time to no avail. Perhaps my past has caught up with me. At the interviews I have attended, it is clear the people who are interviewing me know of my professional past. Or, maybe it is because I am approaching my 61st birthday and ageism that allegedly doesn't exist in the workplace actually does exist. I don't know. I get positive feedback from all of my interviews, yet I am not the successful candidate, why?

My entrenched fear of the bank taking the house has proved to be unfounded. The wolf and I are by now so very well acquainted that I no longer fear being short of money. Our lending institution has been very understanding and with a little bit of robbing Peter to pay Paul, we will make it. We won't be going on any world trips anytime soon, but we will eventually own the house. This beautiful property has kept me going for I would fight to the death for it. It is our sanctuary. Only those who are invited get to cross our threshold. My son has flown the nest and has a family of his own. My daughter is making plans to move out and begin making her own house her home. Since we were married in 1986 my husband and I have had exactly one month where it was just the two of us. Since then, over 32 years later we are preparing for our last chick to leave the nest. Our very beautiful 3/4 acre very soon will be inhabited by just my husband and I.

It is time.

The thing that really makes me sad is that all of us; Margaret, Yanaha, Violet, Meadhbh, Simone and I, all ended up being big losers, be it in health, wealth, marriage or sanity. None of us ever intended to be whistleblowers. The spotlight was unbidden, cast upon us by Narissa who I believe, like us, was a true patient advocate. It was the rabid appetite of the media that saw us all irrevocably changed and punished for truth telling.

I have been a nurse for 50 years. Today, with 5 degrees, I continue to work as a Registered nurse/midwife clinician, this is the only future that Health is prepared to offer me. It has taken me some time to ultimately realise, I don't accept the loss of my career due to my future trajectory being severed by the imposition of a life-time ban on career advancement by NSW Health. My goal of ascension of the nursing hierarchy was on track to gain the experience to be in the running to become Chief Nurse of NSW. We will never know, will we?

I am now 66 years of age and I am known as a damn good nurse. Patients are important to me just as standards of professional practice are.

Today, at the end of my career, I have a position in a nice, peripheral, 'countryish' hospital, where I can positively influence junior nursing staff and promote safe, scientific nursing practice. I plan to work until the house is paid off which will be when I am seventy-eight years old, or dead, whichever comes first.

EPILOGUE

It is 2025 and my story is now told. I once more look forward to the sunrise.

The journey to publication and release of Nurse Blood, for me has been very challenging. NSW Health has been alerted to the existence of the book, who in turn, notified the area health service and my employing hospital. Since that time, a set of circumstances have, I perceive, provided them with a vehicle for the imposition of extreme actions and hardship upon me.

I expected no less.

The Mistress of Darkness is again screeching with laughter, now that my happy thoughts have abandoned me once again.

I must not fear.

Fear is the mind killer...

All of the participants in this book have been appointed pseudonyms. I have written under my own name for I am unrepentant. At times this memoir was pure agony to write as the resurgence of memories pummelled me time and time again, leaving me flat and fearful of failure; that the telling of this story would beat me and the manuscript would never be finished. Often times, months went by without a word being written as I couldn't bear to open the file and face the pain again. This was a very hard story to tell.

There are things now of which I am very sure. I am not a whistleblower, although I have been severely punished for being one. I am a patient advocate.

I no longer resent the term. The difference between being an advocate and being a whistleblower is simply a matter of the escalation of concern. I am a professional nurse who all of my working life has advocated for my patients and have campaigned to improve health outcomes. I applaud my colleagues, the participants in the study for likewise offering their commitment to excellence in patient care. I am also, deeply grateful to them for being brave enough to participate in this research which was gut wrenching for us all. Together, we held fast over a period of eighteen months and three rounds of gruelling interviews that led to the acquisition of our collective truths. We all suffered terribly by reliving those events that have forever changed our lives.

It takes enormous courage to willingly participate in interviews that resurrect and release past demons. I commend my colleagues for their endurance and will forever more be humbled by their truths. I know it came at a terrible cost.

My experience and that of my colleagues must prevail as a lasting legacy to empower all nurses, young and old, to enable them to better understand how a profession such as nursing that is universally admired, can be so destructive. The recommendations as outlined in my PhD thesis are intended to be an instrument for change in healthcare in the state of New South Wales; beginning with the way in which the state reacts to the nurses it employs when they advocate for their patients – regardless of the level of escalation of concern.

It is clear that what nurses advocate for and what the media projects may be two very different things. Once a nurse has exhausted all other avenues of internal reporting, some issues will be significant enough to risk public declaration. It is professional naivety that sees nurses caught up in media storms - lost, unprotected and left wondering when the issue became about them. Nurses must be empowered with the skills and knowledge necessary to escalate patient safety and adverse outcomes with eloquence and scientific, informed expression of the issues of concern. It takes a good deal of confidence and practice to deal with the media. The ability to do so for nurses at least, can only come from universities and healthcare organisations that embrace open disclosure which is demonstrated by strategic media awareness training for staff.

I now live life on my own terms. For the most part, I keep the Mistress of Darkness at bay...for the most part. I am a successful author with three books published, with a work in progress and an established readership. I have given up applying for jobs in

Health because I have found what is a good fit for me work wise and I am happy.

My journey through life as a nurse for the most part has been a privilege, filled with great fun and camaraderie. The profession of nursing however is a hard taskmaster that is not always supportive and its reputation that it eats its own young is well deserved.

I now know all too well that the dark side of nursing is associated with depression, PTSD, bullying, harassment and too often, suicidal ideation. I accept that the last 50 years as a nurse/midwife, has shaped me into the person I am today. I remain committed to 'doing the right thing'. However, I have learned to pick my battles and to step back with a problem is not my responsibility to solve. My daughter always says my moral compass is true, but this life as a nurse/midwife has been a very long, hard road with many bitter lessons learned. It is my fervent hope that this work will be read by members of the general public so they become aware of the risk's nurses take when they advocate to keep them safe. I also hope Nurse Blood becomes a recommended text for university students undertaking any vocation in the social sciences.

Forewarned is forearmed.

From participation comes discovery; a footprint in the future from the voices of our past. To leave a legacy is the most we can hope for.

Kathrine Maree Grover 2025

REFERENCES

Link to PhD thesis: https://rune.une.edu.au/web/retrieve/0c966102-bdf7-40d1-9af6-f619385ff0fd

Page 92: The full ICAC Report can be found online and is readily available to the public: https://www.parliament.nsw.gov.au/tp/files/39438/Report%20into%20allegations%20relating%20to%20the%20former%20South%20Western%20Sydney%20Area%20Health%20Service.pdf

Page 147: The full Peter Garling SC's findings from The Special Commission of Inquiry: Acute Care Services can be found here: https://www.cec.health.nsw.gov.au/__data/assets/pdf_file/0011/258698/Garling-Inquiry.pdf

Inquiry into Complaints Handling Within NSW Health: https://www.parliament.nsw.gov.au/lcdocs/transcripts/1035/120304%20Corrected%20transcript.pdf

GLOSSARY

Health Care Complaints Commission (HCCC)

Independent Commission Against Corruption (ICAC)

South-Western Sydney Area Health Service (SWSAHS)

Central Sydney Area Heath Service (CSAHS)

Senior Executive Services Level 3 (SES 3)

(Extract: Legislative Council - General Purpose Standing Committee No. 2. Complaints handling within NSW Health - Report 8: 17th June 2004)

ABOUT THE AUTHOR

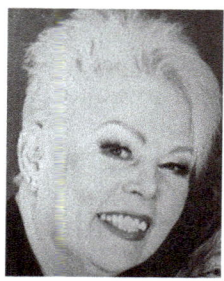

Kathrine Grover
Nurseblood2025@outlook.com

I was born a warrior. My father taught me the meaning of honour and integrity. Life taught me to be a daughter, a mom, a sister, a grandmother and a nurse/midwife. The profession of nursing taught me to value and protect life. Adversity taught me to stand tall, be strong and protect those under my care. I am my father's daughter.

Truth is important to me.

Justice is important to me.

I was born to two middle-class people who were always most at home in the Australian bush. I lived a sheltered, itinerant life, moving from town to town, across states, for my father's work. Over the course of my school life, I attended thirteen different schools—an education in how to fit in.

My mother was a nurse. In 1975, I followed her footsteps to become a Registered Nurse then and a Midwife. I attained two further degrees and a PhD.

My career led me to management, as leading to me is as innate as breathing. What is not innate is failing to report unexpected and adverse patient outcomes. My demand for transparency was not only a career stopper it set me in the sights of the media to be labelled a whistleblower nurse.

I am not a whistleblower but a strong patient advocate who will protect those under my care from harm.

My professional and personal life is forever changed because I chose to tell the truth.

Adverse patient outcomes were made public, and clinical governance was implemented—a high price to pay for justice in healthcare.

In 2025, I remain a truth-teller – and I am unrepentant.

FROM THE PUBLISHER

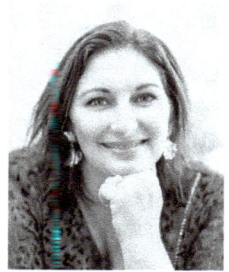

Crystal Leonardi
Bowerbird Publishing
www.crystalleonardi.com

In 'Nurse Blood,' Dr. Kathrine Grover offers a raw, deeply personal account of her 50-year career in nursing and midwifery, inviting readers into the profession's often-hidden emotional terrain.

Kathrine's narrative is captivating as it celebrates the bonds and triumphs that come with a life dedicated to healthcare, while laying bare the profession's systemic issues. Kathrine shines a light on the many nurses' who struggle in silence, highlighting the cost of a profession built on self-sacrifice and care for others.

The title, 'Nurse Blood,' reflects this stark reality, alluding to the literal and metaphorical wounds some nurses endure daily in their commitment to patient care.

'Nurse Blood' is an unmissable read for anyone interested in the human side of healthcare. It reminds us of nurses' powerful impact, even in the face of adversity.

I thank Kathrine for her unbreakable sense of integrity and the legacy she leaves for the next generation of healthcare workers. I also want to take this opportunity to congratulate Kathrine on her unwavering courage and compassionate wisdom. I wish Kathrine all the best.

Defamation Disclaimer: The author and publisher do not intend to defame, harm, or impugn the character or reputation of any individual or entity. Any opinions expressed or events described are not intended to represent or reflect the actions or beliefs of any specific person or group.

No Legal or Professional Advice Disclaimer: This book does not provide legal, medical, financial, or any other form of professional advice. The content is intended solely for informational purposes and should not be construed as advice or a substitute for professional consultation. The author and publisher strongly recommend that readers consult with appropriate professionals regarding any specific issues or concerns they may have.

Accuracy and Reliance Disclaimer: While every effort has been made to ensure the accuracy and reliability of the information in this book, the author and publisher make no guarantees or representations regarding the accuracy, reliability, or timeliness of the content. The information in this book is accurate as of the publication date; however, the author and publisher do not accept responsibility for any errors, omissions, or changes that may have occurred after the book was published. The reader should independently verify any facts or data before relying on them.

No Liability for Actions Taken Based on Content: The author and publisher disclaim any responsibility for any loss, damage, or consequences that may arise from the use or misuse of the information contained in this book. The content is intended for informational purposes only, and any actions taken by readers based on this content are at their own risk. The author and publisher cannot be held liable for any direct, indirect, incidental, or consequential damages resulting from the use of this book.

Factual Accuracy Disclaimer: This book includes factual information and research-based content. However, due to the evolving nature of information, the author and publisher do not guarantee the absolute accuracy of all the facts presented. The author has made every reasonable effort to ensure the reliability of sources and the accuracy of content, but some information may have changed or become outdated. Readers are encouraged to verify the facts independently and consult authoritative sources if needed.

No Endorsement or Affiliation Disclaimer: Any brand names, trademarks, or references to specific products, services, or organizations mentioned in this book are for informational purposes only and do not imply endorsement or affiliation with the author or publisher. The inclusion of these references does not indicate support or sponsorship, and the author and publisher are not responsible for any third-party claims or issues arising from the use of any mentioned products or services.

No Responsibility for External Links Disclaimer: This book may contain references to external websites or online resources. The author and publisher are not responsible for the content, accuracy, or reliability of any third-party websites or materials linked in this book. Links are provided for informational purposes only and do not imply any endorsement of those sites or their contents.

Cultural Sensitivity and Interpretation Disclaimer: The content of this book addresses various cultural, historical, and social issues. While every effort has been made to present these topics with respect and accuracy, interpretations and opinions may differ across cultures and communities. The author and publisher acknowledge that perspectives and interpretations of the information presented may vary and encourage readers to engage with the material thoughtfully.

Update and Revision Disclaimer: The content in this book is based on the best available information at the time of publication. However, due to the constantly evolving nature of knowledge, statistics, laws, and regulations, the author and publisher make no guarantees that the information will remain accurate, up-to-date, or applicable. Readers should be aware that new developments may have occurred since the publication of this book and are encouraged to seek current information from authoritative sources.

www.ingramcontent.com/pod-product-compliance
Lightning Source LLC
Chambersburg PA
CBHW072146070526
44585CB00015B/1013